BS... of Ra... edicine ...nd Surgery

Editor:

Paul A. Flecknell

MA VetMB PhD DLAS DiplomateECVA MRCVS
Comparative Biology Centre, The Medical School
Framlington Place, Newcastle-upon-Tyne NE22 4HH

Published by:

British Small Animal Veterinary Association
Woodrow House, 1 Telford Way,
Waterwells Business Park, Quedgeley,
Gloucester GL2 2AB

A Company Limited by Guarantee in England.
Registered Company No. 2837793.
Registered as a Charity.

A catalogue record for this book is available from the British Library

ISBN 0 905214 46 3

The publishers and contributors cannot take responsibility for information
provided on dosages and methods of application of drugs mentioned in this
publication. Details of this kind must be verified by individual users from the
appropriate literature.

Typeset by: Fusion Design, Fordingbridge, Hampshire, UK

Printed by: Lookers, Upton, Poole, Dorset, UK

ii

Other titles in the BSAVA Manuals series:

Manual of Advanced Veterinary Nursing
Manual of Canine and Feline Behavioural Medicine
Manual of Canine and Feline Emergency and Critical Care
Manual of Canine and Feline Gastroenterology
Manual of Canine and Feline Haematology and Transfusion Medicine
Manual of Canine and Feline Infectious Diseases
Manual of Canine and Feline Nephrology and Urology
Manual of Canine and Feline Wound Management and Reconstruction
Manual of Companion Animal Nutrition and Feeding
Manual of Exotic Pets
Manual of Ornamental Fish
Manual of Psittacine Birds
Manual of Raptors, Pigeons and Waterfowl
Manual of Reptiles
Manual of Small Animal Anaesthesia and Analgesia
Manual of Small Animal Arthrology
Manual of Small Animal Cardiorespiratory Medicine and Surgery
Manual of Small Animal Clinical Pathology
Manual of Small Animal Dentistry
Manual of Small Animal Dermatology
Manual of Small Animal Diagnostic Imaging
Manual of Small Animal Endocrinology
Manual of Small Animal Fracture Repair and Management
Manual of Small Animal Neurology
Manual of Small Animal Oncology
Manual of Small Animal Ophthalmology
Manual of Small Animal Reproduction and Neonatology
Manual of Veterinary Care
Manual of Veterinary Nursing
Manual of Wildlife Casualties

Contents

Contributors

Pip Boydell BVetMed CertVOphthal MRCVS
Animal Medical Centre, 511 Wilbraham Road, Chorlton-cum-Hardy, Manchester M21 0UB, UK

Stephen W. Cooke BVSc MRCVS
Greendale Laboratories Ltd, Lansbury Estate, Lower Guildford Road, Knaphill, Woking,
Surrey GU21 2EW, UK

Barbara Deeb DVM MS
Allpet Veterinary Clinic, Shoreline, WA 98155, USA (Affiliate Professor,
Department of Comparative Medicine, University of Washington, Seattle, WA, USA)

Paul A. Flecknell MA VetMB PhD DLAS DiplomateECVA MRCVS
Comparative Biology Centre, The Medical School, Framlington Place, Newcastle-upon-Tyne NE22 4HH, UK

A. Dermod Malley BA MVB FRCVS
South Beech Veterinary Surgery, 40 Southend Road, Wickford, Essex SS11 8DU, UK

Anna Meredith MA VetMB CertLAS CertZooMed MRCVS
The R(D)SVS Hospital for Small Animals, The University of Edinburgh, Easter Bush, Veterinary Centre,
Roslin, Midlothian, EH25 9RG, UK

Timothy H. Morris BVetMed PhD CertLAS DipACLAM MRCVS
Department of Laboratory Animal Science, SmithKline Beecham Pharmaceuticals,
New Frontiers Science Park, Third Avenue, Harlow, Essex CM19 5AW, UK

Sharon Redrobe BSc BVetMed CertLAS MRCVS
Zoo Veterinary Officer, Bristol Zoo Gardens, Clifton, Bristol BS8 3HA, UK

David H. Scarff BvetMed CertSAD MRCVS
Anglian Referrals, 2 Highlands, Old Costessey, Norwich, Norfolk NR8 5EA, UK

Sally O. Walshaw MA VMD
University Laboratory Animal Resources, Michigan State University, Clinical Center C-100,
East Lansing, MI 48824, USA

David Williams MA VetMB PhD CertVOphthal MRCVS
Department of Clinical Veterinary Medicine, University of Cambridge, Madingley Road,
Cambridge CB3 0ES, UK

Foreword

The staggering rise in popularity of the rabbit kept as a companion animal over recent years has meant that the small animal practitioner has developed an insatiable thirst for knowledge of this area of veterinary medicine. Continuing education courses on rabbit medicine are frequently oversubscribed, despite course provision increasing dramatically. Previously allocated just one chapter in the *BSAVA Manual of Exotic Pets*, the subject now commands a dedicated Manual in its own right.

This is the thirtieth new title produced in the BSAVA Manuals series and stands to be one of the most popular.

The Editor, Paul Flecknell, has gathered together an impressive list of international contributors both from practice and academia. The first two chapters cover handling, restraint, clinical techniques, and general biology and husbandry. The Manual then follows the tried and tested format of a clinically oriented approach in each body system. Chapters on behaviour, therapeutics, anaesthesia, surgical procedures, dentistry and euthanasia round off a comprehensively colour illustrated publication. The book concentrates on the hutch and house rabbit rather than rabbits kept commercially.

This completely new Manual is bound to appeal to veterinary surgeons, veterinary students and veterinary nurses alike and must be an essential addition to every practice library. I am sure that it will also prove equally popular with animal care colleges and interested owners.

P. Harvey Locke BVSc MRCVS
BSAVA President 1999–2000

Preface

The numbers of rabbits kept as pets has increased dramatically, to the extent that they are now the third most popular pet in the UK. This increase in numbers has naturally led to greater demands for veterinary care. This Manual aims to provide a concise guide for the small animal practitioner, but should also be of interest to veterinary nurses, students, and rabbit owners. The contributors have a wide variety of backgrounds, but all share an enthusiasm for this developing area of veterinary medicine, and an interest and affection for rabbits.

Veterinary care of rabbits has of course been established for many years, but has been predominantly oriented towards treatment of laboratory rabbits and rabbits reared for human consumption. The spectrum of conditions seen in pet rabbits differs from those seen in these other groups, and the emerging popularity of house rabbits has increased the importance of behavioural problems. The authors have specifically tried to address the management of the pet rabbit, although much of the material will have relevance to other rabbit groups.

One major difficulty encountered when writing this book was the relative lack of controlled clinical trials of specific therapies in pet rabbits. In addition, relatively little data are available concerning pharmaceutical agents. It is hoped that this situation will improve rapidly as the veterinary profession and the animal health industry begin to meet the challenges posed by these animals.

As Editor, I would like to thank the contributors for their help, cooperation and encouragement in the production of this manual, and the editorial staff at BSAVA for their efforts, especially in speeding the publishing timetable for the book. Staff at the University of Newcastle provided much valuable help, both in manuscript processing and providing illustrations. Finally, thanks are due to my wife, Ruth, for tolerating my editorial activities – especially at Christmas!

Paul A. Flecknell
March 2000

CHAPTER ONE

Handling, Restraint and Clinical Techniques

Dermod Malley

INTRODUCTION

Clinical assessment of the pet rabbit begins, as in the examination of all species, with the collation of an adequate case history. A suggested format of questions is illustrated in an Appendix at the end of this chapter. Particular attention should be paid to the two main factors that affect the health of the pet rabbit: nutrition and stress.

Nutrition is discussed in Chapter 2. The clinician must understand this important subject and the functioning of the lagomorph digestive system (see Chapter 5) to be fully able to assess the rabbit patient.

Stress may be defined as an animal's response to intrusion. Intrusive factors or stressors may vary from terrifying predators or mildly irritating vermin to chronic nutritional abuse or even lack of shelter from a prevailing wind. In acute situations, a physiological chain of events is manifested (see Figure 1.1) which leads to the 'flight or fight' response. In situations of chronic stress the corticosterone receptors of the hypothalamic–pituitary axis are saturated and the negative feed-back mechanism becomes blocked, allowing excessive corticosterone production by the adrenal glands. The resultant increase in, and sustained maintenance of, blood corticosterone levels leads to the increased risk of establishment of chronic infections so commonly encountered in the pet rabbit.

Rabbits are very nervous, sensitive animals with a low pain threshold and require firm, but gentle handling.

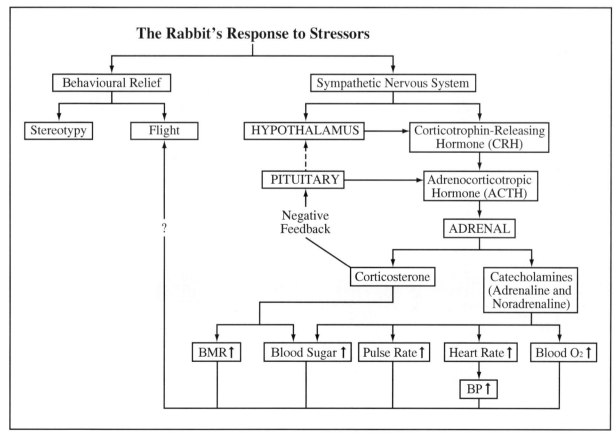

Figure 1.1: *The physiological chain of events in the stress response.*

OBSERVATION

The rabbit should be observed in quiet circumstances. Minimal stimulus will cause the animal to freeze and press itself against the table top. Flicking fingers and vibrant 'kissing' noises are inappropriate, as these encourage the animal to become tense rather than to relax. Background noises such as road traffic, rushing practice personnel, ringing telephones, slamming doors and barking dogs all prevent the rabbit from relaxing. However, once the animal does relax it shows its inquisitive nature, and then observation can begin. The eyes should be prominent and bright, the ears erect (except in lop-eared breeds), and the nose should twitch rhythmically.

If the animal is being observed in its own quarters the faeces should be inspected, size and consistency of the pellets being particularly important. Scanty small faecal pellets may indicate anorexia or gastrointestinal disturbance.

HANDLING, RESTRAINT AND CLINICAL EXAMINATION

Rabbits are best transported to the surgery/clinic in an enclosed box or cat carrier. Most clinicians prefer to approach the boxed animal from above as many rabbits will crouch downwards in response to a vertical approach whereas a horizontal approach may encourage the animal to defend itself and bite or scratch the handler. However, great care must be taken to stop the animal from leaping in the air from a top-opening box or carrier. Draping a towel over the open top of the box may be a sufficient deterrent.

The rabbit skeleton is relatively fragile, comprising only 7–8% of bodyweight compared to 13% in the cat. Care must be taken at all times to support the delicate caudal lumbar spine which can easily be fractured by careless restraint. To achieve this, the author prefers to grasp by the 'scruff' of the withers and to lift the animal from the carrier, supporting the rump with the other hand (Figure 1.2). The rabbit is then placed on a non-slip rubber surface on the consulting room table and restrained by the assistant who covers the eyes with one hand and the rump with the other (Figure 1.3). The back is now examined for parasites and the presence of skin disease. The assistant lifts his/her fingers to allow the clinician access to the tail or 'scut'.

To allow access to the head, the assistant places the hands on each side of the chest with the thumbs on the withers, the fingers curved around the front legs and the palms on the sides of the chest, supporting the sides of the body with the forearms (Figure 1.4). The ears (both sides of the tragus) and eyes can now be examined by the clinician. Particular attention must be paid to the lacrimal apparatus by applying digital pressure which will express pus (if any is present) from the ampulla as shown in Figure 1.5. Bacteriological examination of ocular discharges is often required and a small-tip swab, previously moistened in sterile saline, can be introduced into the conjunctival fornix to obtain a sample.

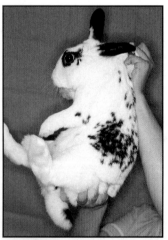

Figure 1.2: It is vital to support the weight of the animal at the rump.

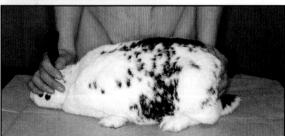

Figure 1.3: With the rabbit on a non-slip surface, one hand over the eyes and another over the rump provides safe and adequate restraint.

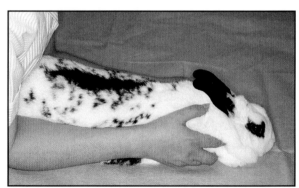

Figure 1.4: Access to the head with the body adequately restrained.

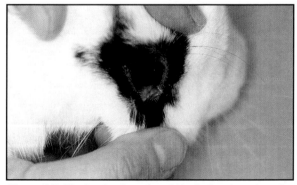

Figure 1.5: The lacrimal punctum is in the lower conjunctiva quite far from the palpebral margin.

Auscultation of the thorax is performed with the rabbit restrained as shown in Figure 1.3. Due to the presence of fur, a bell-ended stethoscope is used to avoid the adventitious sounds produced by movement against the fur.

At no time should the animal be left unrestrained on the table, as the flighty nature of the species means that it may attempt to jump to the floor, with disastrous results. Very little clinical detail can be acquired by single-handed restraint and examination.

The clinician then takes over from the assistant, lifts the animal by the scruff of the withers (Figure 1.6), supports the rump with the other hand and turns the animal over on to its back until it is lying along the left forearm, while the rump is held by the upper arm against the chest (Figure 1.7). If the animal is likely to struggle, the head may be restrained by gently including the ears in the grip on the scruff of the withers. Restraining a rabbit in dorsal recumbency disorientates it and produces a hypnotic state.

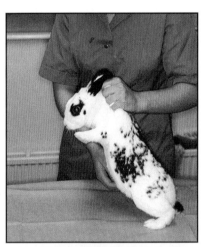

Figure 1.6: The rabbit is lifted from the table prior to turning it over on its back.

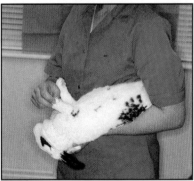

Figure 1.7: Restraint with the rabbit in dorsal recumbency and the rump secured against the handler's chest.

The incisors may now be examined by dilating the philtrum. The molars can be palpated intraorally with the fourth finger in a tractable animal trusted not to bite, or an attempt may be made to visualize them with an otoscope. The author uses a halogen-illuminated light metal otoscope for this purpose, having sacrificed plastic specula to the nibbling action of rabbit's teeth in the past. To examine the molars, buccal cavity and tongue adequately, it is necessary to open the mouth with a gag, dilate the buccal cavity with a pouch dilator

(Figure 1.8) and deflect the cheeks with a spatula. This requires deep sedation or general anaesthesia (see Chapter 12). Inspection of the dewlap of the adult doe is important because of the high incidence of intertrigial dermatitis in this area. Predisposing causes include leaking water (sipper) bottles and excessive salivation due to overgrown teeth.

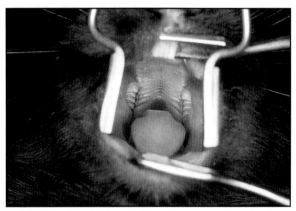

Figure 1.8: Examination of the teeth can be achieved only with the mouth opened with a gag and the buccal cavity dilated with a suitable implement. A spatula can be used to separate the cheek from the back teeth.

The ventral aspect of thorax and abdomen is now examined and palpated. The nipples of does should be examined for the cystic enlargement indicative of uterine disease; the vent, prepuce, vulva (see Figure 1.9) and the bilateral perineal clefts should also be examined for crusts indicative of treponematosis or *Psoroptes cuniculi* mite infestation.

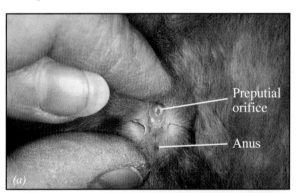

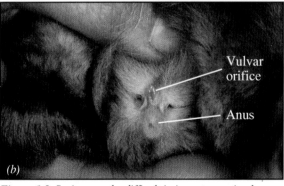

Figure 1.9: Sexing may be difficult in immature animals (before testicular descent in the male). (a) The preputial orifice is always circular. (b) The vulvar orifice is elliptical. The anogenital distance is longer in males than in females.

At this point it is convenient to examine the feet and perhaps clip the animal's claws (Figure 1.10). The fore legs may also be conveniently examined while the animal is being restrained on its back. The medial aspects of the fore feet must be examined for dried pus or mucus obtained by wiping a discharging nose or weeping eye. Particular attention should be paid to the nail beds as they are so well covered in fur that lesions are easily overlooked.

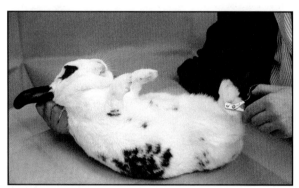

Figure 1.10: Restraint in dorsal recumbency on a non-slip surface is safest for claw-clipping.

The rectal temperature may be recorded at any stage of the examination but obviously the information gained is more significant if this is carried out at the beginning of the procedure. The thermometer is inserted with the animal in dorsal recumbency; it must be remembered that the anal canal of the rabbit is directed dorsally.

The animal is now passed to the assistant who supports the thorax with the back against his/her own chest. One hand holds the chest with the fore legs restrained between the fingers. The palm of the other is passed caudally down the abdomen and the thighs are gently held between thumb and forefinger and third and fourth fingers and pushed caudally until the hips are fully extended (Figure 1.11). The first, second and third fingers are gently curved under the vent. The clinician examines the ventrum for the presence of ectoparasites, hair loss and skin disease, and percusses the abdomen, principally to detect caecal resonance (Figure 1.12). In a rabbit normally fed on a high fibre diet, resonance is restricted to an area occupying '10 to 12 o'clock' in the right epigastric area. Rabbits fed on a highly fermentative, high starch, low fibre diet have a resonance that occupies a much larger area (often '8 to 3 o'clock'). Disease states leading to an increased liquidity of caecal contents result in a markedly reduced resonance, reminiscent of balloting a rubber hot-water bottle full of water. Obese animals produce muffled sounds on abdominal ballotment. Displacement of the resonant area indicates enlargement of one or more abdominal viscera.

With the rabbit still restrained in this upright position, the clinician can palpate the ventral aspect of the mandible and inspect the nostrils for discharge (which may also be reflected in the presence of dried mucus on

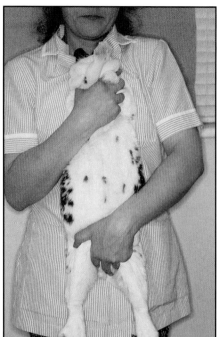

Figure 1.11: Safe restraint of the rabbit for visual inspection of the ventral abdomen and ballotment of the abdominal contents.

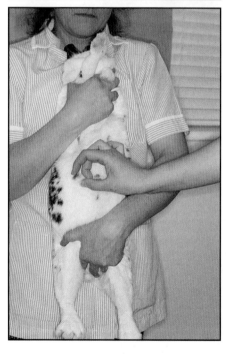

Figure 1.12: Detection of caecal resonance.

the medial aspect of its ipsilateral carpus). The hind legs are examined in this position. The hips, stifles, hocks and digits are extended and flexed in turn, the assistant changing his/her grip on the lower abdomen to accommodate this manipulation. The clinician should be aware that lateromedial stability of the rabbit's patella is less than that of dogs or cats.

It is extremely important to weigh the animal and to record the weight on each examination, especially if it is hospitalized. Variations in weight are often the only clinical parameters on which the progress of a case can be assessed. Some animals will sit quietly on a table-top digital scales, but others may have to be placed in a box of known weight.

RESTRAINT OF THE FRACTIOUS RABBIT

Often the only way to restrain a particularly nervous rabbit is to lift it cleanly and firmly by the scruff of the withers and swing it under the other arm, trapping it against the lower ribcage, as shown in Figure 1.13.

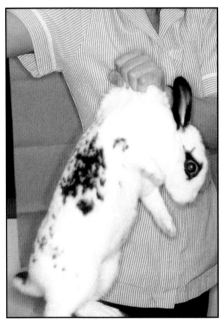

Figure 1.13: Swinging a fractious rabbit under the arm.

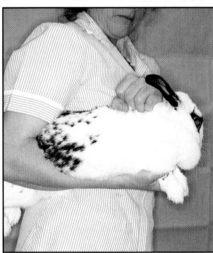

COLLECTION OF BLOOD SAMPLES

Marginal ear vein

Blood samples can be obtained easily from the marginal ear vein in most rabbits, but the vein can be markedly constricted in dehydrated animals, or in rabbits housed in cool temperatures, and it may be extremely small in many pet animals, notably dwarf breeds. The hair overlying the skin must be shaved with clippers or a scalpel before the vein is easily visualized. Most rabbits make a sudden movement as the vein is entered, but this can be prevented by the prior use of EMLA cream (Astra Zeneca) (see Chapter

12). Withdrawal of blood is aided if an assistant compresses the vein near the base of the ear. Some workers state that, in healthy rabbits, sedation and analgesia can be provided by the use of fentanyl/fluanisone (0.2–0.3 ml/kg i.m.) (Hypnorm, Janssen Cilag) or acepromazine (0.5 mg/kg) plus butorphanol (1 mg/kg) (both i.m., see Chapter 12). These drug mixtures cause vasodilation of the ear vein, as well as analgesia and sedation, and so facilitate venepuncture. The technique of placement of an 'over-the-needle' catheter in the ear vein is illustrated in Chapter 14.

Jugular vein

Blood samples are obtained from the jugular vein by restraining the animal on a non-slip surface at the table edge with the neck extended and the jaw raised. The fore legs are extended below the table top. The side of the neck is clipped and access to the jugular vein is achieved (Figure 1.14). Sedation may be required in advance of this procedure, the author's preference being diazepam (1 mg/kg i.m.) 20 minutes before venepuncture. It is often difficult to visualize the vein, but it is usually simple to palpate it. This procedure is similar to that performed daily in cats by small animal veterinary surgeons.

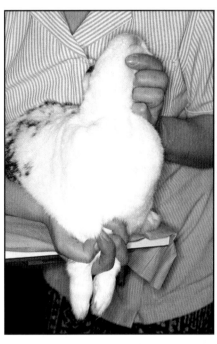

Figure 1.14: Access to the jugular vein.

Cephalic vein

The cephalic vein is approached by restraining the animal on a non-slip surface in sternal recumbency, raising the vein with a tourniquet before exposure by clipping.

Femoral vein

Access to the femoral vein is achieved by restraining the animal in lateral recumbency with the target leg slightly extended. The medial aspect of the thigh is

clipped distally to the stifle and pressure is applied to
the femoral vein in the inguinal canal (Figure 1.15).
The femoral vein is very mobile in rabbits and must be
stabilized with the thumb. The application of local
anaesthesia (EMLA cream) or use of benzodiazepines
may be necessary.

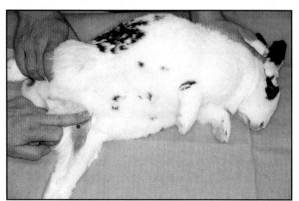

*Figure 1.15: Lateral restraint to gain access to the femoral
vein. Note this vein is extremely mobile and difficult to
stabilize for venepuncture.*

Auricular artery
The central auricular artery is frequently used by
clinicians for so-called intravenous injections and blood
sampling with disastrous results, as the procedure can
lead to ischaemic necrosis of most of the pinna. It is,
however, a convenient means of obtaining samples for
arterial blood gas analysis, and for placement of an
'over-the-needle' catheter for monitoring arterial pressure during anaesthesia (see Figures 12.12 and 12.13).
Care must be taken to apply pressure to the artery for
several minutes to avoid haematoma formation after
removal of the catheter or needle.

Size of needles used
Generally, 23 G (0.6 mm) or smaller needles are used
in venepuncture of the jugular and marginal ear vein,
depending on the size of the rabbit and the experience
of the operator, but 25 G needles (0.5 mm) are used in
other veins. Fur may be clipped with an electric clipper
or simply removed by plucking. The skin is cleaned
with alcohol (isopropyl alcohol) or antiseptic (povi-
done–iodine or chlorhexidine).

URINE COLLECTION

To obtain urine by cystocentesis the rabbit may be
restrained by an assistant in the same manner as for
percussion of the abdomen as described above, except
that the rump is supported from behind and the clinician holds the rabbit's hind leg with the thumb on the
medial aspect of the thigh. The needle is directed at an
angle of 20–30 degrees to the inguinal canal towards
the bladder (see also Chapter 13). Alternatively, it is
often quite simple to express urine from the bladder

directly into a universal container. Catheterization of
the urethra is very difficult in both sexes and is said to
cause urethrospasm in bucks. If it is necessary to
catheterize a buck, premedication with dipyrone/
hyoscine (Buscopan, Boehringer Ingelheim), at 0.25
ml/kg s.c.may be required.

COLLECTION OF FAECES

Faeces should be assessed macroscopically for size of
pellet and fibrous content. Saturated saline is the
flotation medium of choice for examination of the
faeces for the presence of coccidian oocysts. *Saccha-
romyces* sp. (yeasts) are frequently encountered
symbionts of the rabbit caecum and counts in excess of
3 million per gram of faeces are frequently encountered. In the author's experience, rabbits receiving oral
antibiotics frequently show more than 300 million/g,
and often have to be treated with antimycotic agents
(e.g. nystatin) to control softening of the stools.

COLLECTION OF SKIN AND FUR

Skin scrapings are seldom required in rabbit medicine.
Cheyletiella and *Leporacarus* spp. of mites are identified on plucks and brushings of rabbit fur. Full details
are given in Chapter 9.

ADMINISTRATION OF MEDICATION

Prior to administration of medication to pet rabbits, the
clinician must ensure that there is adequate restraint of
the patient; this is very important as many individuals
are much less phlegmatic than those kept in laboratories or commercial units. Their response to injections
and attempts at oral administration of medications is
certainly far less predictable. Poorly restrained animals are likely to leap without warning from the
examination table, often with disastrous results.

Oral medication
It is very easy to administer small (<2 ml) amounts of
fluids to rabbits, which will readily lick drops from a
needleless hypodermic syringe placed in the diastema.
The syringe is gently applied to the philtrum and
passed back to the diastema.
   Larger quantities of fluids are administered orally
by the author by the use of a cut-off piece of tubing
from an intravenous infusion giving set pushed on to
the luer adapter of an injection syringe. The free end of
the giving set is flamed to soften the plastic and remove
any sharp edges. Alternatively, an infant feeding tube
can be used, but this is less suitable for feeding liquid-
ized diets with a high fibre content. The compliant
rabbit may be restrained by an assistant, as in Figure

1.4, and the clinician restrains the head, although some animals will allow a clinician to dose single-handed. The clinician's hand is placed over the poll, the fingers and thumb engaging the maxillary bones on each side. The tube is sparingly lubricated with KY Jelly (Johnson and Johnson) and the free end is placed into the philtrum, moved to one side of the incisors and passed into the cranial oesophagus (Figure 1.16). With practice, an experienced clinician can learn to avoid the incisors which otherwise sever the tube. This technique is particularly useful for the administration of alfalfa slurry to anorectic animals.

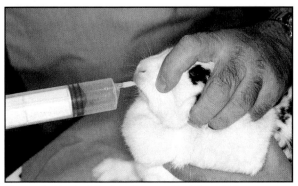

Figure 1.16: Oral feeding ('gavage') of the rabbit.

Naso-oesophageal tubes are also useful for oral fluid therapy (see Figure 1.17) and are introduced as follows:

1. Additional holes are made in the caudal aspect of an FG 5–8 feeding tube. The distance from external nares to the caudal end of the sternum is measured and marked on the tube with tape or a pen.
2. Local anaesthetic drops are applied to the nostrils or the tube is lubricated with xylocaine gel. After 3–5 minutes local anaesthesia should be adequate for the tube to be moved without resistance or discomfort.
3. The rabbit is restrained in sternal recumbency on the non-slip table top and the head is elevated.

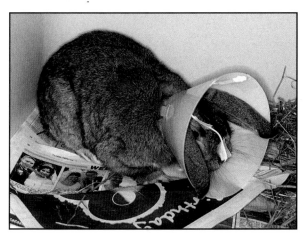

Figure 1.17: Naso-oesophageal tube in place.

4. The lubricated tube is placed in the ventral nasal meatus directing it medially and ventrally. The rabbit's head is returned to the normal flexed position as the pharynx is approached so that the tube passes gently down the oesophagus.
5. *Proper placement is assessed by radiography.* Assessing the site of the caudal end of the tube by injection of saline is not appropriate as the rabbit does not always cough when the saline (or tube) is placed in the trachea. The distal end of the tube may be found to be in the stomach and should be withdrawn to a position in the caudal oesophagus.
6. The tube is sutured or glued to the head of the rabbit (over the bridge of the nose and at the base of the ears). An Elizabethan collar is fitted only if the animal interferes with the tube.
7. The blended food is strained prior to administration and the tube is flushed with water after administration. Administering blended caecotropes may be attempted but may not be necessary as caecotrophy (and feeding) should be possible with the tube in place. Caecotrophy is obviously not possible when the animal is wearing an Elizabethan collar.

Parenteral medication

Intramuscular, subcutaneous and subconjunctival injections are all administered with the animal restrained in the sternal position by an assistant with the hands of the assistant over the eyes and the rump of the rabbit as described above.

Subcutaneous injections

These are given into the dorsal aspect of the thorax in the 'scruff' but not over the abdomen and never into the ventral aspect of thorax or abdomen. The skin of rabbits is surprisingly tough and difficulty is often experienced puncturing the skin. Care should be taken to ensure that the needle penetrates the skin at a wide angle and that the lumen of the needle is directed properly under the skin. The maximum volume of a subcutaneous injection given to a rabbit is dependent on the size of the animal and the irritancy of the product. Up to 30 ml of isotonic fluid per kilogram of bodyweight can be given on each side of the animal when providing fluid therapy.

Intramuscular injections

These are given in the quadriceps muscles. The skin over the muscle must be tensed firmly prior to injection. The maximum volume of a non-irritant solution that can be given to rabbits is of the order of 0.3–0.5 ml/kg, depending on the breed. This fact tends to dictate the route of administration when there is a choice between subcutaneous and intramuscular routes. It is also possible to administer an intramuscular injection single-handed to a pet rabbit if the animal is restrained under the arm on a table (see Figure 1.18).

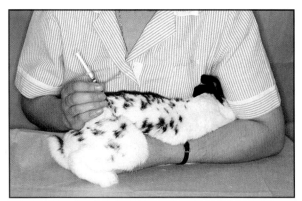

Figure 1.18: *Single-handed intramuscular injection of the rabbit.*

Subconjunctival injections

These are required quite often in pet rabbits, as conjunctivitis following suppurative dacryocystitis is a very common occurrence in these animals. The use of ophthalmic local analgesia is advised prior to subconjunctival injection. The rabbit is restrained as shown in Figure 1.3 or 1.4 and the injection is administered into the bulbar conjunctiva in the same manner as in dogs. The volume administered varies from 0.25–0.50 ml.

Intraosseous injections

Intravenous cannulation is described in Chapter 12, but this author's preferred approach for fluid therapy is the use of spinal or intraosseous needles in the tibia or femur. The trochanteric fossa of the femur or the cranial edge of the tibial crest is located by digital palpation. The area is clipped, cleaned and disinfected. A spinal or intraosseous needle is introduced gently but firmly with or without prior administration of a local anaesthetic and the needle is passed into the intramedullary cavity.

Intrathoracic injections

This is the route preferred by the author for euthanasia of torticollis, terminal myxomatosis or pneumonia cases in which restraint leads to asphyxia and unnecessary stress. The needle is inserted between two ribs and allowed just to enter the pleural cavity. The movement of the lungs encourages the rapid absorption of the euthanasia agent by the pleura.

Intradermal injections

As Shope's fibroma vaccine is given by this route to vaccinate against myxomatosis, intradermal injection is a common procedure in rabbits. The point of a 27/29 G needle is engaged in the skin perpendicularly and the barrel of the syringe is lowered so that the needle can be passed into the skin. Vaccine manufacturers tend to recommend the hairless area of the base of the pinna for this procedure, but any area of the back may be used if the fur is clipped (not plucked in order to avoid the possibility of the reaction of the poxvirus in epilated skin) (Figure 1.19).

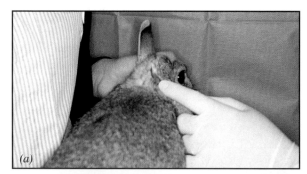

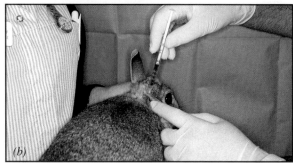

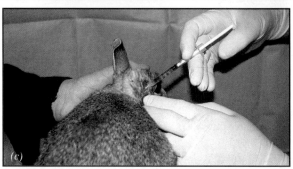

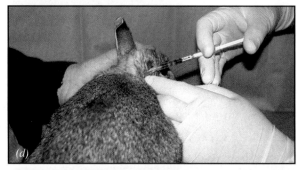

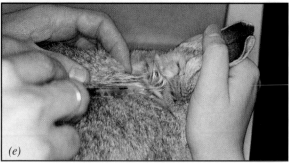

Figure 1.19: *(a) Selection of site for intradermal injection. (b) The point of the needle is inserted to engage the skin at right angles to the epidermis. (c) The barrel of the syringe is lowered through 90 degrees, keeping the point of the needle engaged as above. (d) The needle is advanced parallel to the surface of the skin, truly intradermally. (e) Close up view of the needle in situ.*

Intraperitoneal injections

These are given in the inguinal quadrant with the rabbit restrained vertically (Figure 1.20). The needle is passed parallel to the inguinal canal and the plunger withdrawn to make sure that the urinary bladder has not been punctured.

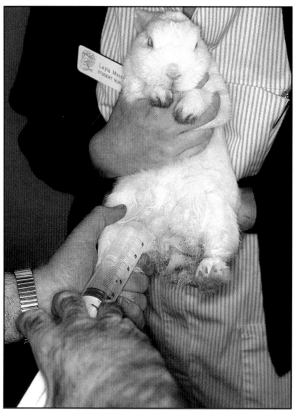

Figure 1.20: Intraperitoneal fluid administration.

Topical medication

Ophthalmic drops

These are instilled directly on to the globe. The rabbit must be fully restrained against the handler's body and the upper eyelid controlled by digital pressure on the skin dorsal to the upper eyelid. An assistant is required to retract the lower eyelid if it is necessary to apply fluid eye drops to the lower conjunctival fornix.

Ear drops

These must be applied to both sides of the tragus of the auricular canal so that the blind-ended intertragic incisure is treated properly.

Topical skin preparations

Applications of oil-based topical skin preparations are inappropriate because of deleterious effects on the fine fur of the rabbit. In general, for the treatment of dermatoses, the author prefers detergent-based products which are thoroughly rinsed and dried afterwards.

Other routes

The use of enemas and emetics is inappropriate.

REFERENCES AND FURTHER READING

British Veterinary Association Animal Welfare Foundation, Practical Animal Handling, 1, Small Mammals, VHS format videotape, available from BVAAWF, 7 Mansfield Street, London, W1M 0AT

Burgmann PM (1991) Restraint techniques and anaesthetic recommendations for rabbits, rodents and ferrets. *Journal of Small Animal Exotic Medicine* **1**, 73–78

Fowler ME (1995) Laboratory rodents and rabbits. In: *Restraint and Handling of Domestic Animals, 2nd edn,* pp. 176–178. Iowa State University Press, Ames.

Harkness JE (1987) Rabbit husbandry and medicine. *Veterinary Clinics of North America – Small Animal Practice* **17** (5), 1019–1030

Hillyer EV (1994) Pet rabbits. *Veterinary Clinics of North America – Small Animal Practice* **24** (1), 25–39

Mader DR (1997) Basic approach to veterinary care. In: *Ferrets, Rabbits and Rodents; Clinical Medicine and Surgery,* ed. EV Hillyer and KE Quesenberry, pp. 160–168. WB Saunders, Philadelphia

Malley AD (1994) The pet rabbit in companion animal practice: 1. A clinician's approach to the pet rabbit. *Irish Veterinary Journal* **47**, 9–16

Malley AD (1995) The pet rabbit in companion animal practice: 2. Clinical general examination. *Irish Veterinary Journal* **48**, 307–311

Malley AD (1996a) The pet rabbit in companion animal practice: 3. Special examinations. *Irish Veterinary Journal (incorporating Irish Veterinary Times)* **49**, 112–114

Malley AD (1996b) The pet rabbit in companion animal practice: 5. The administration of medicine. *Irish Veterinary Journal (incorporating Irish Veterinary Times)* **49**, 407–410

Stein S and Walshaw S (1996) Rabbits. In: *Handbook of Rodent and Rabbit Medicine,* ed. K Laber-Laird *et al.,* pp.187–190. Pergamon, Oxford

Appendix 1.1 over the page ▶

Owner details

Owner's name .... Date ....

Address ....

....

Telephone numbers (home) .... (work) ....

Rabbit details

Name of rabbit ....

Breed ....

Colour ....

Age/Date of birth ....

Sex ....

Neutered?   Y/N

Site/address where rabbit is kept (if different) ....

....

Date acquired ....

Source: pet shop/friend/breeder (delete as appropriate) or other ....

Do you keep other rabbits?   Y/N   If yes please give details:

Name	Breed	Date acquired	Source	Any illnesses?

Details of other pets

Do you keep other pets?   Y/N   If yes please give details:

Species	Date acquired	Source	State of health	Closely associated with rabbit?

Indoor ('House') rabbits

Does your rabbit have access to the whole house?   Y/N

If confined to one room please give details ....

What is the temperature? ....

Is it double glazed?   Y/N   Centrally heated?   Y/N

Has the rabbit damaged any household items?   Y/N

Please give details:

Item	How damaged	When (date)

Appendix 1.1: Clinical history questionnaire for rabbit owners.   ▶

Indoor ('House') rabbits continued

Is your rabbit kept in a hutch indoors?   Y/N

If yes please give approximate dimensions: height: ....   depth: ....   width: ....

Describe the bedding and litter in the hutch ....

....

Are there smokers in the house?   Y/N

Is there an indoor boiler?   Y/N

If so, when was it serviced last? .... (date)

Is your rabbit allowed access to the garden?   Y/N   *If yes, please complete the section on Outdoor rabbits*

Is this supervised?   Y/N

Where does your rabbit urinate and defaecate? ....

Do you use litter?   Y/N   *If yes, please describe* ....

Outdoor rabbits

Where is the hutch situated? .... Does it face north/south/east/west? ....

Are there overhanging trees?   Y/N   Is there shelter from vermin or predators?   Y/N

Have you ever seen rats, mice, foxes, cats or birds of prey in your garden?   Y/N

Please describe the vegetation in the garden ....

Does your rabbit drink from a bowl or a sipper-bottle? ....

What is the litter on the floor of the hutch? ....

All rabbits
Bedding

Do you use straw/hay/both? .... What is the type (species) of straw or hay? ....

Food

Describe the rabbit's diet. ....

Please list all the items he/she is known to eat and the quantities of these items if possible ....

....

Where do you buy your rabbit's food?

a) Pet shop; b) Supermarket; c) Pet superstore; d) Greengrocer; e) gather it or grow it yourself;

f) other (please describe) ....

Do you use processed food?   Y/N

If so, please name it ....

Do you buy it packed or loose? ....

Have you changed the diet recently?   Y/N

If yes, please state when and give a description of the previous diet ....

....

Do you give: vitamins   Y/N

minerals   Y/N

tonics   Y/N

medicines   Y/N

probiotics?   Y/N

If so, please name and state the way you give them ....

Water

How much water does your rabbit drink each day? ....

Has the drinking increased or decreased? ....

If increased when did you notice this? ....

Grooming

How often do you groom your rabbit? ....

Do you use a brush, comb, a cloth or just your hand? ....

Appendix 1.1 continued: Clinical history questionnaire for rabbit owners.   ▶

General information

When did your rabbit: moult? ....

breed? ....

nest? ....

have phantom pregnancy? ....

mate? ....

Does he/she dig or burrow?   Y/N

Any previous problems?   Y/N

Please state with dates: ....

The present problem

Please describe your rabbit's clinical signs (symptoms) ....

Is the nose twitching normally?   Y/N   Any nasal or ocular discharge?   Y/N

Any excessive drinking?   Y/N

Do you notice coprophagy (rabbit eats droppings)?   Y/N

Are the droppings normal in appearance and size?   Y/N

When did you first notice any difference in the number and size of the droppings? ....

Does your rabbit spray urine?   Y/N   What colour is the urine? ....

Has this increased/decreased lately? .... If so, please give date of change ....

Does your rabbit thump?   Y/N

Has this increased/decreased lately? .... If so, please give date of change ....

Is the skin/fur normal?   Y/N   Is there excessive scratching?   Y/N

Any odd positioning or loss of use of any limbs?   Y/N   *If yes, please describe* ....

Any abnormal vocalization?   Y/N

Appendix 1.1 continued: Clinical history questionnaire for rabbit owners.

CHAPTER TWO

General Biology and Husbandry

Anna Meredith

INTRODUCTION

The domestic rabbit *Oryctolagus cuniculus* originated from the European wild rabbit. There are many other species of rabbit which, along with cottontails, pikas and hares, make up the Order Lagomorpha. Man's relationship with the European or 'true' rabbit was first recorded by the Phoenicians over 1000 years BC, when they named the Iberian peninsula *i-shephan-im* (literally 'the land of the rabbit'), which the Romans converted to the Latin form, *Hispania*, and hence the modern word Spain.

The wild rabbit has long been hunted but it is unclear when domestication first took place. The Romans kept rabbits in walled enclosures (*leporaria*) and there is evidence that they brought the rabbit to Britain, although they did not survive in the wild at this time. In Europe, and especially France, the domestication process was well under way by the fifth century AD, and in the twelfth century the Normans brought rabbits to Britain, where they became established and remain as both a domestic and wild animal. Man introduced the rabbit throughout the world, often with devastating effect; for example, the absence of predators in Australia and New Zealand led rabbits to become pests. The rabbit has not, however, become established in the wild in North America.

With domestication of the rabbit came the development of different breeds and varieties (colours). All domestic rabbits are the same species as the wild European rabbit. In 1995, a total of 61 breeds and 531 varieties of rabbit were recognized in the UK (Figure 2.1), and more are constantly evolving by selective breeding and mutation, although most pet rabbits are cross-breeds. In the UK, breeds are currently divided into Fancy (e.g. Himalayan, Flemish, Netherland Dwarf), Fur (e.g. Chinchilla, Beveren, New Zealand) and Rex (mainly different coat colours and patterns with basic rex fur type) categories. In the USA, classification of breeds differs, and links to a useful series of websites illustrating US breeds can be found at USA American Rabbit Breeders Association (http://members.aol.com/arbanet/arba/web/photo.htm). In the UK, the British Rabbit Council has its own website (http://www.thebrc.fsnet.co.uk/), which includes the judging standards for each breed, and a growing number of illustrations.

Over the centuries, man has used the rabbit for food, sport, clothing, as a scientific model and a hobby (the rabbit 'fancy'). The keeping of rabbits as pets developed in Victorian times and their popularity has grown enormously, to the point where rabbits are now the third most popular mammalian pet in the UK. Although traditionally kept, and thought of, as a children's pet, increasing numbers of rabbits are kept by adults and as house pets, becoming as much a part of the family as the more traditional cat or dog.

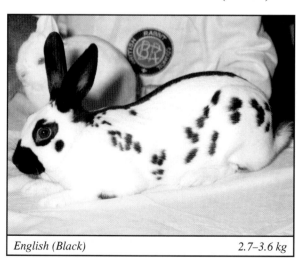

English (Black)	2.7–3.6 kg

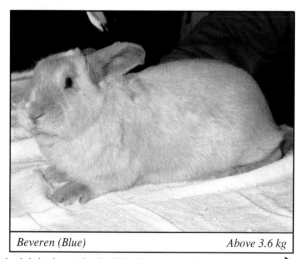

Beveren (Blue)	Above 3.6 kg

Figure 2.1: Examples of breeds of domestic rabbit, showing typical adult bodyweight. © CBC, University of Newcastle.

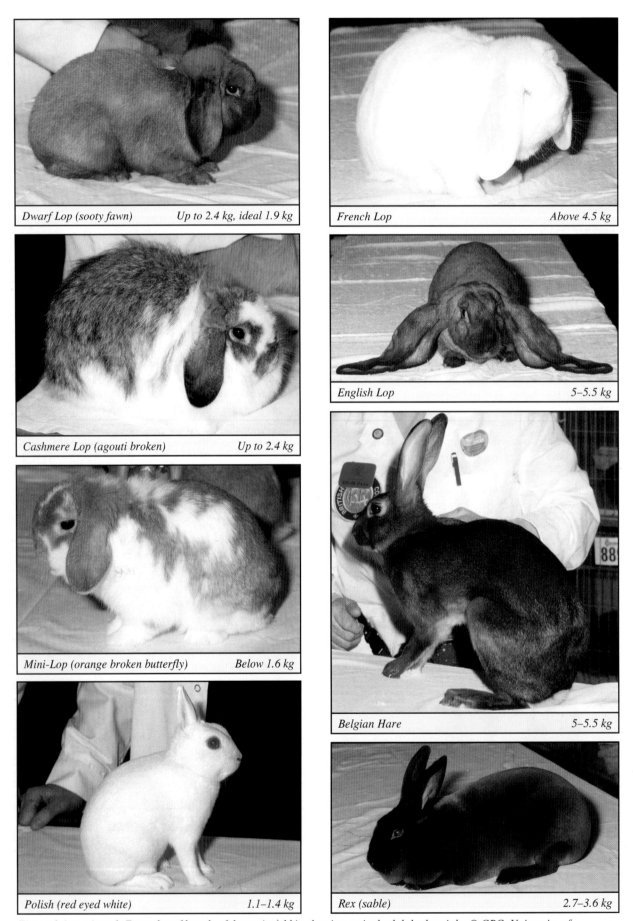

Figure 2.1 continued: Examples of breeds of domestic rabbit, showing typical adult bodyweight. © CBC, University of Newcastle.

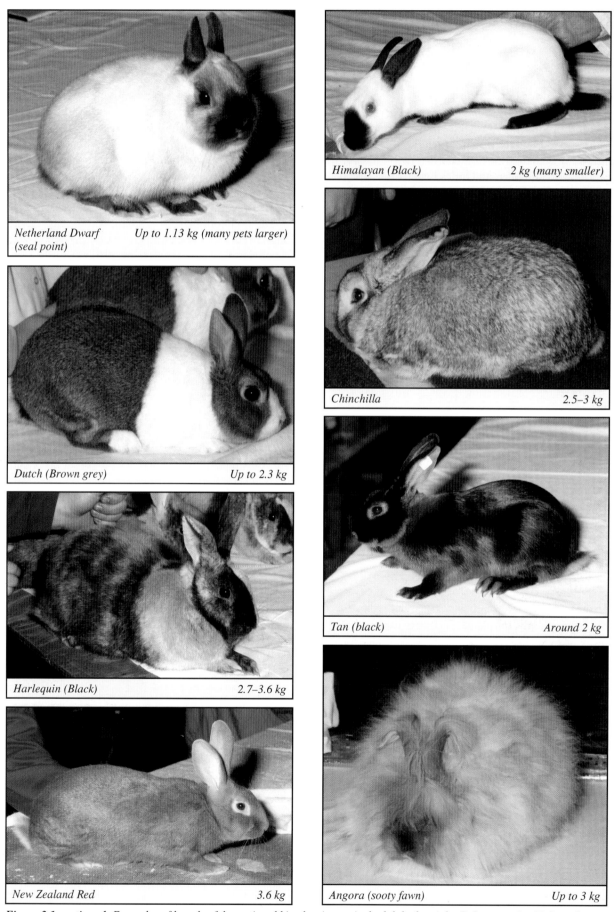

Netherland Dwarf   Up to 1.13 kg (many pets larger)
(seal point)

Dutch (Brown grey)   Up to 2.3 kg

Harlequin (Black)   2.7–3.6 kg

New Zealand Red   3.6 kg

Himalayan (Black)   2 kg (many smaller)

Chinchilla   2.5–3 kg

Tan (black)   Around 2 kg

Angora (sooty fawn)   Up to 3 kg

Figure 2.1 continued: *Examples of breeds of domestic rabbit, showing typical adult bodyweight. © Comparative Biology Centre, University of Newcastle. Photographer: Don Wright.*

RABBIT ANATOMY AND BIOLOGY

Rabbits are social burrowing herbivores that are natural prey for a large number of carnivores. As a prey species they have evolved to be constantly vigilant, lightweight and fast moving, with a highly efficient digestive system that enables them to spend the minimum time possible above ground, thus reducing the danger of capture. Likewise, to avoid attracting the attention of predators, rabbit behaviour is not florid and overt and relies heavily on scent (see Chapter 10).

Most rabbits live for 5–8 years, but some individuals live to 10 years or more (Figure 2.2).

Heart rate	180–300 beats per minute
Respiratory rate	30–60 breaths per minute
Body temperature	38.5–40.0 °C
Daily food consumption (pellets)	50 g/kg/day
Daily water consumption	50–15 ml/kg/day
Daily urine production	10–35 ml/kg/day
Adult bodyweight (breed dependent)	1–10 kg
Newborn kitten body weight	30–80 g
Life expectancy	5–10 years

Figure 2.2: Physiological data for the rabbit.

Musculoskeletal system
The rabbit skeleton is light, making up only 7–8% of bodyweight. The front limbs are short and fine, in contrast to the long and powerful hindlimbs. From the tarsus distally, the plantar surface of the hindlimb is in contact with the ground at rest. The spine is naturally curved. Bodyweight ranges from 1 to 10 kg and conformation varies depending on the breed, from the squat or 'cobby' shape of the dwarf breeds to the lithe and lean 'racy' Belgian Hare. In some breeds, skull morphology can lead to disease, especially dental problems. For example, some dwarf breeds have a mandibular prognathism that causes incisor malocclusion, and breeds with a foreshortened skull seem predisposed to nasolacrimal duct and dental problems.

Great care must be taken when handling rabbits. Osteoporosis is often present owing to lack of exercise and low calcium intake, and a kick from the powerful hind legs can result in the rabbit fracturing its lumbar vertebrae (usually L6/L7). The vertebral formula of the rabbit is C7T12L7S4C16 although in some animals there are 13 thoracic vertebrae. The forelimb has five digits and the hindlimb four. Rabbit muscle appears light pink.

Dentition and the oral cavity
The rabbit has a cleft upper lip. The dental formula is 2/1 0/0 3/2 3/3. The incisors are used for grazing, and food is then passed to the back of the mouth for grinding. The incisors have an enamel layer only on the anterior surface, which wears more slowly than the posterior surface thereby maintaining a chisel shape for cutting herbage. The vestigial second pair of upper incisors is located directly behind the first pair; these are known as 'peg teeth.' All teeth are open rooted and long crowned and grow continuously. The cheek teeth are wider apart on the maxilla than on the mandible, and the lower teeth grow faster than the upper.

The oral commissure is small, and the oral cavity long and curved. Cheek folds across the diastema make visualization of the cheek teeth difficult in the conscious animal. The tongue is large and has a mobile rostral portion and a relatively fixed thicker caudal portion (torus). There are four pairs of salivary glands: parotid, submaxillary, sublingual and zygomatic.

Skin and fur
Female rabbits have a large fold of skin under the chin known as the dewlap, from which they pull hair to line the nest before kindling. The toes and metatarsal areas are completely covered with hair, and there are no footpads. Scent glands are located on the underside of the chin, either side of the perineum (inguinal glands) and at the anus (anal glands). The inguinal glands are large and pouch-like and often contain a yellow-brown oily deposit.

Hair coat depends on breed. The normal coat consists of a short soft undercoat protected by longer guard hairs. The only hairless areas are the tip of the nose, part of the scrotum and the inguinal folds. In the Rex breed the guard hairs are shortened and so do not protrude above the level of the undercoat. Satin breeds have an altered hair fibre structure that gives the coat a characteristic sheen. Angora rabbits have a very long undercoat and guard hairs (harvested for spinning into wool), which need regular grooming to prevent matting.

The guard hairs are the first to emerge in newborn kittens, followed by the undercoat. After a few days this soft baby coat is well developed, and it persists until about 5 or 6 weeks of age. An intermediate or pre-adult coat then replaces this, followed by the adult coat by about 6–8 months of age. Thereafter most rabbits moult twice a year (spring and autumn), but this can vary. Moulting starts at the head and proceeds caudally. Pregnant or pseudopregnant does undergo a loosening of the hairs on the belly, thighs and chest, which are then easily plucked to line the nest and expose the nipples. Does possess four or five pairs of nipples on the ventrum. Nipples are absent in the male.

Tactile vibrissae are present on the muzzle and are used to help locate food and orient the rabbit when underground.

Eyes and ears

The large eyes are located laterally, with a very wide field of vision to aid detection of predators. Rabbits have a blind spot in the area beneath the mouth, so food is detected by the sensitive lips and vibrissae. The lens is large and almost spherical, and the ciliary body is poorly developed, so accommodation is limited. The retina is merangiotic, with the optic disc lying above the midline of the eye and retinal vessels spreading horizontally out from it. The optic disc has a natural depression or cup. There is no tapetum lucidum.

A third eyelid is present and the Harderian gland is located just behind it. This gland has two lobes, the upper being white and the lower larger and pink. The gland is larger in males, especially during the breeding season. The orbital venous sinus is very large in the rabbit, and great care must be taken during enucleation to avoid damaging it and causing serious haemorrhage (see Chapter 13).

The nasolacrimal duct has a single lacrimal punctum in the medial aspect of the lower eyelid. From here there is a short (about 2 mm) canaliculus coursing medially and ventrally into a funnel-shaped lacrimal sac, supported medially by the lacrimal bone. The duct then enters the maxilla through a semicircular foramen in the lacrimal bone. The duct has two sharp bends as it courses towards the nose, proximally in the maxillary bone and at the base of the incisor teeth (Figure 2.3). The duct narrows at these points – the duct epithelium is undulating, and the opening into the nasal meatus is very small, which makes the nasolacrimal duct prone to blockage.

The ears are highly vascular with large arterio-venous shunts, and they are involved in heat regulation. Ear size varies between breed, and those animals with ears that hang down are referred to as 'lops'.

Digestive tract

Rabbits are hindgut fermenters, adapted to digest a low-quality high-fibre diet consisting mainly of grass. However, unlike other similar fermenters such as the horse, the rabbit has a very rapid gut transit time and eliminates fibre from the digestive tract as soon as possible. This permits body size and weight to remain low, which is advantageous in a prey species. In the wild, feeding takes place mainly in the early morning, evening and at night.

The gastrointestinal tract (Figure 2.4) makes up 10–20% of bodyweight.

Stomach

The stomach is thin walled and poorly distensible, with a well developed cardia and pylorus. Vomiting is not possible in the rabbit. Food and caecal pellets are always present in the stomach.

Intestine

The duodenum and jejunum are narrow, and at the end of the ileum there is the sacculus rotundus, also known as the ampulla ilei or ileocaecal tonsil, a structure that is rich in lymphoid follicles.

Caecum

The caecum is very large, thin walled and coiled and has many sacculations (or haustrae). It terminates

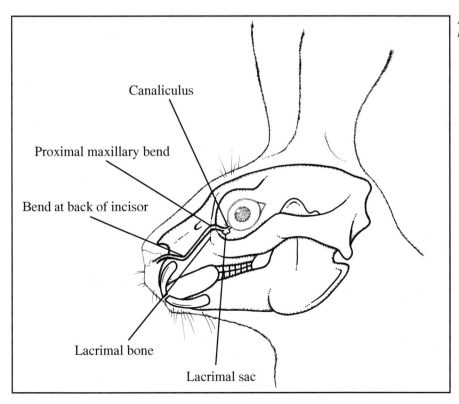

Figure 2.3: The anatomy of the nasolacrimal duct in the rabbit.

Canaliculus

Proximal maxillary bend

Bend at back of incisor

Lacrimal bone

Lacrimal sac

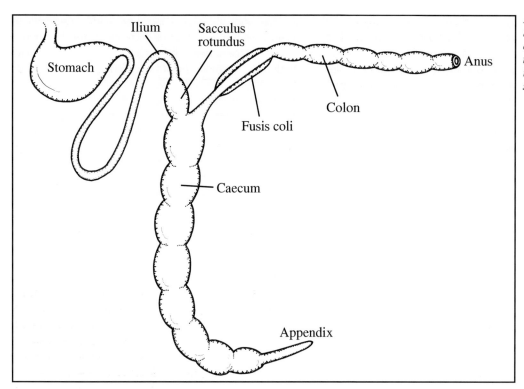

Figure 2.4: Schematic diagram of the anatomy of the digestive tract in the rabbit (not to scale).

in the vermiform appendix, which is also rich in lymphatic tissue. The caecum lies on the right side of the abdomen. Caecal contents are normally semifluid.

Antiperistaltic waves move fluid and non-fibrous particles back into the caecum for fermentation. Three to 8 hours after eating, and thus mainly at night, soft mucous-covered caecal pellets are expelled and eaten directly from the anus (a process known as caecotrophy, coprophagy, refection or pseudorumination). Arrival of the caecotrophs at the anus triggers a reflex licking of the anus and ingestion of the caecotrophs (see Figure 2.5), which are swallowed whole and not chewed. A muscular band of richly innervated tissue with a thickened mucosa, the fusis coli, lies at the end of the transverse colon and acts to regulate colonic contractions and controls production of the two types of pellets.

The most prevalent caecal bacteria are of the anaerobic Gram-negative genus *Bacteroides*. Gram-negative ovals, fusiform rods, large ciliated protozoans (*Isotrichia*) and yeasts (*Cyniclomyces guttulatus*) are also present. Coliforms are not present in healthy rabbits.

The mucous covering protects the caecal pellet bacteria from the low pH of the stomach. Caecotrophs remain in the stomach for up to 6 hours with continued bacterial synthesis, and eventually the mucus layer dissolves and the bacteria are killed. This process of caecotrophy allows absorption of nutrients and bacterial fermentation products (amino acids, volatile fatty acids and vitamins B and K) and the redigestion of previously undigested food. A food item thus passes twice through the digestive tract in 24 hours.

Colon
The colon is sacculated and banded. Colonic contractions separate fibrous from non-fibrous particles, and fibre moves rapidly through for excretion as hard faecal pellets (Figure 2.5).

	Dry matter	Crude protein	Crude fibre
Faeces	53%	15%	30%
Caecotrophs	39%	34%	18%

Figure 2.5: Composition of faeces and caecotrophs.

Liver, pancreas and gall bladder
The pancreas is diffuse and located in a pocket formed by the transverse colon, stomach and duodenum. The liver has four lobes and a gall bladder is present. Rabbits secrete mainly biliverdin in the bile rather than bilirubin. The pancreatic duct and the bile duct are separate.

Spleen
The spleen is flat and elongated and lies on the dorso-lateral surface of the greater curvature of the stomach.

Respiratory system
Rabbits are nose breathers (mouth breathing is a very poor prognostic sign). In a normal rabbit the nose moves up and down 20–120 times a minute ('twitching'), but this will stop when the rabbit is relaxed or anaesthetized. The glottis is small and visually obscured by the back of the tongue. Reflex laryngospasm is common in the rabbit, which can complicate endotracheal intubation. The thoracic cavity is small, and

breathing is mainly diaphragmatic. The lungs have three lobes, and the cranial lung lobes are small (left smaller than right). Large amounts of intrathoracic fat are often present. The thymus remains large in the adult rabbit and lies ventral to the heart, extending into the thoracic inlet.

Cardiovascular system

The heart is relatively small and lies cranially in the thoracic cavity. The right atrioventricular valve has only two cusps. The rabbit aorta has neurogenic rhythmic contractions.

Urinary system

Rabbit kidneys are unipapillate. Renal function is discussed further in Chapter 6.

Urine

Urine is the major route of excretion for calcium. Serum calcium concentrations in rabbits are not maintained within a narrow range, but depend largely on dietary intake, with excess excreted via the kidney. Rabbit urine is often thick and creamy owing to the presence of calcium carbonate crystals. It can also vary in colour from pale creamy yellow through to dark red (often mistaken for haematuria by owners), due to the presence of porphyrin pigments thought to be derived from the diet.

Reproductive system

Does have no uterine body, two separate uterine horns and two cervices opening into the vagina. The vagina is large and flaccid. The mesometrium is a major site of fat deposition. The placenta is haemochorial.

Bucks have two hairless scrotal sacs either side of and cranial to the penis. There is no os penis. The inguinal canals remain open throughout life.

RABBIT HUSBANDRY

Housing

Rabbits are traditionally kept outdoors in a hutch (Figure 2.6) but can also be kept indoors as a house pet ('house rabbit'; Figure 2.7).

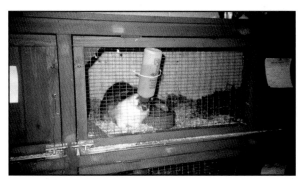

Figure 2.6: Traditional rabbit hutch, which is often too small.

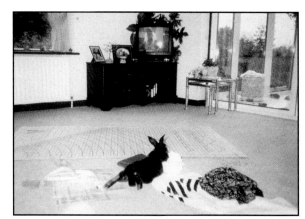

Figure 2.7: Rabbits are increasingly kept as house pets ('house rabbit'). Courtesy of Sally Machell.

Hutches

Hutches available from pet shops are usually too small, certainly as the sole accommodation for a rabbit. Hutches for pets are invariably made of wood, although laboratory rabbits are kept in ones made of metal and plastic. Wood has the advantage of being cheap but can be gnawed. It also can absorb urine and thus may smell if there is insufficient bedding or cleaning is infrequent. Hutches of various designs are available (Figure 2.8), but the essentials are a dry draught-free secluded nest area and an area for exercise. A solid-fronted nesting area and mesh-fronted living area are usually provided.

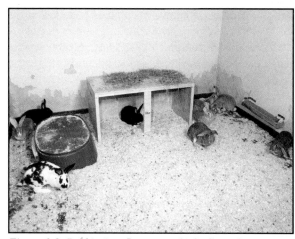

Figure 2.8: Rabbits in a floor pen, which allows for exercise and greater expression of normal behaviour.

Hutches should always be as large as possible with, at the very least, sufficient room for the rabbit to stretch up fully on its hindlimbs and to stretch out. If confined to the hutch for long periods, the rabbit should be able to perform at least three 'hops' from one end to the other. Exhibition rabbits are often kept in sheds with banks of wooden hutches stacked in three tiers. The bottom hutch should be at least 20 cm above the floor. Litter boards can be placed across the bottom of the opening of the hutch to prevent bedding falling out when the door is opened.

Outdoor hutches should be raised off the ground and protected from wind and rain. A felted roof sloping toward the back is suitable, as are louvred shutters that can be closed in particularly inclement weather. Direct sunlight should be avoided as heat stress and heat stroke occur easily in rabbits. Rabbits cannot sweat and do not increase water intake when hot. Rabbits tolerate cold better than heat, and as they do not have brown fat deposits they shiver when very cold. Good ventilation is essential to prevent respiratory disease.

Bedding
Bedding must always be provided – a layer of newspaper or wood shavings (not sawdust) plus straw, or straw alone. Laboratory rabbits prefer to sit on straw rather than shavings.

Water and food
Water bottles can be attached to the outside of the mesh front with a wire clip. Ceramic or metal feeding bowls are most hygienic and will not be gnawed, and hay can be fed loose or dispensed from a rack or net. Wire mesh hay racks can be used to divide adjacent hutches. Food hoppers and automatic water valves are often used for large groups and in commercial or laboratory situations.

Hygiene
Cleanliness is essential to prevent disease, and hutches should be cleaned at least once a week. Wet soiled bedding can cause ulcerative plantar pododermatitis ('sore hocks,' see Chapter 9), and high ammonia levels predispose to respiratory disease. Outdoor rabbits must be checked every day, with special attention paid to the perineal area in summer months as caking of caecotrophs or sitting in wet soiled bedding can predispose to myiasis ('flystrike,' see Chapter 9). Lack of caecotrophy and caking of caecotrophs in this area is often erroneously interpreted as diarrhoea. The cause can be obesity, spinal pain or dental disease.

Exercise area
An exercise area must always be provided in addition to a hutch. This can be in the form of a mobile run, ark or permanently fenced area of grass (Figure 2.9). Alternatively, a shed or garage can be used to provide a floor pen. Raised shelves or platforms are readily used. If rabbits are housed outside it should be remembered that does dig deep burrows, and measures to prevent escape should be taken, such as paving the edges of the pen or sinking wire mesh below ground level. Rabbits can jump well; covering the run or pen with a mesh top will prevent escape, as well as providing protection from potential predators such as cats and dogs. Due to their natural prey status, rabbits should always be provided with appropriate 'bolt holes,' such as empty cardboard boxes or pieces of drain pipe, to use if alarmed (see Figure 2.9).

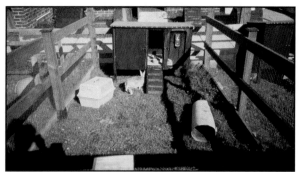

Figure 2.9: *A rabbit in a run on grass, with bolt holes for shelter.*

Contact with wild rabbits should be prevented to minimize the risk of disease transmission by direct contact (e.g. viral haemorrhagic disease) or vectors such as the rabbit flea (e.g. myxomatosis), and suitable fly and mosquito control should be considered in summer months.

House rabbits
House rabbits should have a secure cage area where they can be restrained when the owner is absent. Wire cages with plastic bases are suitable. Exercise around the house should be encouraged. Rabbits naturally urinate and defecate in one place and thus are easily trained to use a litter tray by repeatedly placing them in the tray on acquisition. It may be necessary initially to place some droppings in the tray. Wood- or paper-based litter should be used, as Fuller's earth products can be harmful if ingested. Electrical cables must be protected from chewing, and poisonous house plants such as *Dieffenbacchia* avoided. Chewable toys are enjoyed by house rabbits, e.g. cardboard boxes, old telephone directories, commercial cat or bird toys. House rabbits will readily learn to use 'cat-flaps' for access.

Companions
Rabbits are social animals and should be provided with a companion wherever possible. Littermates can be kept together but should be neutered if of opposite sexes. Unrelated females will usually tolerate each other if sufficient space is provided, but they can fight. Introduced intact bucks will fight and inflict severe injuries. All introductions should be supervised, and neutering will minimize the risk of conflicts.

Rabbits are often kept with guinea-pigs, but this is not advisable as bullying by the rabbit can occur. If they are kept together, guinea-pigs should be provided with an area that is inaccessible to the rabbits. It should be remembered that rabbits can harbour *Bordetella bronchiseptica*, which is pathogenic in guinea-pigs.

Other house pets can be well tolerated, but dogs and cats should not be left unsupervised with rabbits.

Farmed rabbits
Commercially farmed rabbits are kept very differently from pets, mainly in single-tier systems with mesh

floors and no bedding. The MAFF Code of Recommendation for the Welfare of Rabbits (1987) recommends minimum cage sizes. Laboratory rabbits are kept either individually in cages or in groups in floor pens, in accordance with strict hubandry and welfare guidelines, e.g. the Animals (Scientific Procedures) Act (1986) in the UK. Bedding and various devices for environmental enrichment are increasingly used.

Diet

In the wild, rabbits are essentially grazers, although they will forage on leaves and shoots at low level. The composition of grass is about 20-25% crude fibre, 15% crude protein and 2-3% fat. Commercial rabbit diets are often too low in fibre and too high in protein, fat and energy. Indigestible fibre (lignocellulose) stimulates gastrointestinal motility and has a protective effect against enteritis. Diets low in fibre and high in available carbohydrate cause caecocolic hypomotility, prolonged retention of digesta, increased volatile fatty acid production and adverse alterations in pH and microflora. This leads to digestive disturbances, including diarrhoea, especially around the time of weaning. The energy requirements of a rabbit can be met very rapidly on a concentrate diet, compared with the situation in the wild, where most of the animal's time above ground is spent feeding. Feeding a concentrate diet can lead to dental disease owing to lack of wear, obesity and boredom-associated problems such as stereotypic behaviour and aggression. In addition, many rabbits are selective eaters and leave the grass pellet component of a commercial mix, favouring the grains and pulses. These favoured items are low in calcium, and this can lead to bone and dental disease (see Chapter 13).

The best diet for a rabbit is grass and good quality grass hay (e.g. Timothy grass), with a small amount of a good quality high-fibre (18-24%) commercial diet with protein levels around 15%. Alfalfa hay can be given, especially to growing animals, but care should be taken if alfalfa pellets are also fed, as alfalfa is high in calcium and large amounts in the diet could predispose to urolithiasis. Fresh vegetables and small amounts of fruit can also be provided, but fruits high in simple sugars should be avoided. Commercial rabbit mixes, consisting of pulses, grains, grass pellets and biscuits, should not be fed *ad libitum*, as this leads to selective feeding and obesity. A rabbit in good condition should have palpable ribs and vertebrae. Hay should always be available (Figure 2.10) and can be fed from racks or nets to increase time spent feeding. The importance of hay in maintaining gastrointestinal and dental health cannot be overemphasized. Carrots or other vegetables can be suspended from the cage roof to act as an edible toy and to increase the time spent eating.

Sudden changes in diet should be avoided, as should frosted or mouldy food and lawnmower clippings. Rabbits enjoy sweet foods, but sugar-rich

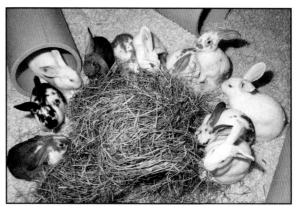

Figure 2.10: *Hay or grass is essential to maintain gastrointestinal and dental health, and should make up most of the diet.*

treats should not be fed (although they may be of use in tempting an anorexic animal to feed or when training an animal to reinforce desirable behaviour (see Chapter 10)).

Kittens show interest in solid food at about 2 weeks of age, and coprophagy starts at about 3 weeks of age. Stomach pH in non-weaned kittens is 5.5-6.0, but this decreases to 1.0-2.0 after weaning. Coprophagy usually commences 3-8 hours after feeding.

Water intake is fairly high, at about 10% of body weight. Drinking bottles are easier to keep clean than water bowls and they avoid wetting of the dewlap, which can lead to a moist dermatitis (see Chapter 9).

BREEDING

Sexual maturation

Onset of puberty depends on breed but is at around 4-5 months of age in the female and 5-8 months in the male. Within a breed, does tend to be slightly larger than bucks but bucks have broader heads. Smaller breeds mature earlier than larger ones. Does tend to be more territorial than bucks; to avoid aggression the doe should be taken to the buck or to neutral territory for breeding.

Rabbits are reflex ovulators. There is no definitive oestrous cycle, but periods of receptivity usually occur for 12-14 days, followed by 2-4 days of non-receptivity while new follicles are developing. This can, however, be highly variable, and some does will become receptive every 4-6 days during the breeding season (January to September).

Mating behaviour

When receptive, a doe becomes very active, rubs her chin on objects and exhibits lordosis, and the vulva becomes congested and reddish-purple. Sexually mature bucks will mate at any time.

Courtship behaviour is brief (about 30 seconds) and involves sniffing, licking and following the doe. Enurination - the spraying of a jet of urine at the doe - is common sexual behaviour. Copulation is very brief and involves a vigorous thrusting intromission, which often leads to the buck falling backwards or sideways and vocalizing. Ovulation occurs 10 hours after copulation.

Does may also mount each other, and this or an infertile mating can induce ovulation and lead to a pseudopregnancy, which lasts about 18 days.

Pregnancy

Pregnancy can be detected by palpation 2 weeks after a successful mating. Normal gestation is 30–32 days. Passive immunity is acquired by placental transfer before birth. Nest-building behaviour involves burrowing if possible, and pulling of fur from the dewlap, flanks and belly to line the nest and expose the nipples.

Parturition

Parturition usually occurs in the early morning. Litter size varies between 4 and 12 kittens, with the larger breeds producing larger litters. The kittens are altricial.

Neonatal care

Rabbit milk is exceptionally nutritious, and nursing is for only a few minutes once, or occasionally twice, a day. This brief nursing period is often misinterpreted by owners as mismothering, but is entirely normal. The parental bond is maintained by scent, with the doe marking her kittens with her chin and inguinal gland secretions. Handling of the kittens can lead to mismothering, and so this should be avoided, particularly during the first week of the kittens' lives. Kittens emerge from the nest at about 2–3 weeks of age and can be weaned at 4–5 weeks of age. Early handling and socialization is important in pet rabbits.

IDENTIFICATION

For exhibition purposes, rabbits are permanently marked with metal rings placed around the hind leg just above the tarsus. Some breeders use one side for bucks and the other for does, but there is no requirement for a particular side. In the UK rings are sold only by the British Rabbit Council and are available in 10 different sizes appropriate for the various breeds (Figure 2.11). Ring numbers are registered against the purchaser, and if the rabbit is sold, the ring number is transferred to the new owner. Rabbits without rings are automatically disqualified from exhibition. Tattooing on the inside of the ear can also be used to identify rabbits.

BEHAVIOUR

Rabbit behaviour is significantly different from that of cats and dogs owing to their prey status. They have poor display of greeting behaviour, pain and fear. Scent is much more important than sight, and each animal has an

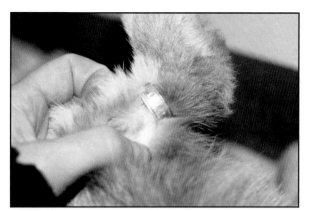

Figure 2.11: *A rabbit identification ring correctly placed above the tarsus.*

individual scent profile. They can distinguish between familiar and unfamiliar humans, and between men and women. Socialization of young rabbits is often overlooked. Kittens emerge from the nest at about 2 weeks of age and are weaned at 4–5 weeks old, but are generally not homed, and therefore handled to any great extent, until about 6–8 weeks of age.

Rabbits are highly social. In the wild they live in warrens usually containing 70 or more individuals, but groups are broken down into 2–8 individuals. Foraging takes up most of the time in the wild, in the early morning and at night. Rabbits should not be kept singly unless the owner can devote a lot of time to them, but should rather be housed in neutered groups or pairs. They spend a lot of time engaged in mutual grooming and lying together. Does are more territorial than bucks, and as they reach sexual maturity may become aggressive towards the owner and other animals. Does may also bite, dig and chew flooring and household items, spray urine and mount other rabbits (see Chapter 10). If outdoors on soil the doe may excavate deep tunnels.

A well socialized pet rabbit will beg for treats, 'hum' at and circle the owner, stand on its back legs and lick the owner's hands and arms. They are inquisitive and enjoy exploring. Picking up objects with the teeth and throwing them is also common, as is exploratory chewing (beware of electrical cables).

A rabbit in pain will be immobile with a hunched posture, and may grind its teeth and show increased aggression. Thumping with the hind leg is an alarm call. Fear elicits either complete immobility or a flight response, with often frantic attempts to escape, which can be accompanied by screaming.

Rabbits have not been bred for positive behaviour traits, and behavioural problems are not uncommon (see Chapter 10). Individual rabbits have distinct 'personalities,' which can range from extremely timid to very aggressive. In general, the smaller breeds tend to have a more nervous disposition. Aggression is generally learnt, i.e. the owner leaves the rabbit alone if it behaves aggressively. Other causes of aggression are territorial behaviour, boredom, pain, improper socialization and negative association, i.e. a previous aversive or traumatic situation. Behavioural aggression can be successfully treated in many cases using similar techniques to those used in dogs (see Chapter 10).

REFERENCES AND FURTHER READING

Manning PJ, Ringler DH and Newcomer CE (1994) *Biology of the Laboratory Rabbit, 2nd edn.* Academic Press, San Diego

BVAAWF/FRAME/RSPCA/UFAW Joint Working Group on Refinement (1993) *Laboratory Animals Refinements in Rabbit Husbandry* **27**, 301–329 (2nd report)

Cheeke PR (1987) *Rabbit Feeding and Nutrition.* Academic Press, London

Harcourt-Brown FM (1996) Calcium deficiency, diet and dental disease in pet rabbits. *Veterinary Record* December 7 **139**, 567–571

McBride A (1998) *Why Does My Rabbit...?* Souvenir Press, London

Sandford JC (1996) *The Domestic Rabbit, 5th edn.* Blackwell Science, Oxford

USEFUL ORGANIZATIONS

The British Houserabbit Association, PO Box 346, Newcastle-upon-Tyne NE99 1FA (http://www.houserabbit.co.uk/)

The British Rabbit Council, Purefoy House, 7 Kirkgate, Newark, Nottingham NG24 1AD (http://www.thebrc.fsnet.co.uk/)

The American Rabbit Breeders Association, PO Box 426, Bloomington, IL 61702, USA

CHAPTER THREE

Clinical Chemistry and Haematology

Stephen W. Cooke

INTRODUCTION

The investigation of disease in any animal may be frustrated by a lack of clinical information that can be easily obtained and is cost-effective, owner-'friendly' and relevant to the case. This is more so in the 'exotic' species. As rabbits are considered as being 'exotic' pets, any assistance that augments the clinician's efficiency should be eagerly grasped. Blood testing has recently gained popularity in general practice due, in part, to the introduction of in-house analysers. In addition, more clinicians are appreciating that the intelligent use of haematology and biochemical information will assist them in providing a better veterinary service to their patients.

BLOOD SAMPLING

Volumes

The blood volume of a healthy rabbit is between 5.5 and 7% of its bodyweight. Up to 10% of total blood volume may be safely removed at any one time, provided the animal is in good health (and a maximum of 25% of the blood volume may be removed over a 2-week period).

A 1.0 ml blood sample is more than enough for a complete blood count (CBC) and 1.5 ml of serum (3 ml of whole blood) is sufficient for most diagnostic laboratories to carry out a very comprehensive biochemistry profile. Carrying out an in-house glucose estimation (using one of the human diabetic dry chemistry analysers, which are quite capable of producing clinically valid results) will obviate the need for filling a fluoride-oxalate tube and will save 0.5–1.0 ml of blood. The 4 ml of blood required may be safely taken from a rabbit as small as 700 g. If smaller haematology sample tubes are available (check with a commercial laboratory for such specialist supplies), then a 0.4 ml sample will suffice for the CBC (especially if an air-dried blood smear is made at the time of venepuncture and submitted with the rest of the sample) and a 533 g rabbit may then be sampled with confidence.

Sites and techniques

A nail clip technique should not be used for rabbits; it is painful for them, contaminates the sample with tissue debris, may prematurely clot blood in sample tubes (and thus wastes time as well as blood) and may lead to secondary nail infections. The marginal ear vein and cephalic, jugular or lateral saphenous veins are all accessible and easy to use for obtaining diagnostic samples. Details of the techniques are given in Chapter 1.

Cardiac puncture is used in experimental facilities but is not to be recommended in general practice due to the obvious risks involved. Historically, the marginal ear vein has been made more prominent and blood flow increased by the use of xylene. However, this chemical is irritant (and possibly carcinogenic) and must be removed with spirit after the blood has been taken; its use is thus in question at present. Petroleum jelly is a better alternative. Using finger pressure as a tourniquet also increases blood flow.

A fine (22–25G) hypodermic needle is introduced into the vein and blood collected directly from the needle hub into the tubes. Rabbit blood coagulates relatively quickly and will form a clot if not mixed with the anticoagulant during collection (this may not be easy in practice). Attaching a syringe and using minimal back-pressure will allow more speedy collection and prevent this problem but many animals will struggle if the vein is irritated when the syringe is attached, thus dislodging the needle. This can be avoided by prior application of EMLA cream (see Chapter 1). A butterfly set may help to avoid this problem but has a dead volume (as well as irritant weight) of its own; if used, it should be primed with anticoagulant first (heparin only as EDTA will greatly elevate potassium levels if allowed to contaminate the heparin or serum tubes destined for biochemistry analysis).

HAEMATOLOGICAL EVALUATIONS

Submission of blood samples

Tubes

Sample tubes available for use are 0.4–1 ml with EDTA (violet or pink tops). It is important to fill the tube with the correct volume of blood (to the line) as EDTA modifies some parameters if present in the wrong concentration.

Smears

A very useful addition for haematological examinations (and one which is often much appreciated by clinical haematologists) is the submission of one or more air-dried blood smears made at the time of venepuncture. A properly made smear will allow for the accurate assessment of red and white cell morphology, which may have been lost or modified during the time it takes a sample to reach an external laboratory.

Complete blood count

The CBC comprises:

- Total white cell count
- Differential white cell count (which should be reported as the absolute numbers of each cell population as well as percentages of each)
- Comment (or lack of it if all parameters are considered by the examining haematologist to be within normal limits)
- Red cell parameters (see below).

At this point it should be noted that a proper microscopic examination of a stained blood smear is infinitely more valuable than a simple mechanical report from an analyser. It would be naive to assume that white and red blood cell counts alone (even if augmented by an instrument's three-part white cell differential) could provide information about the important cytological appearance of each cell type and the likely significance. Conditions such as leukaemias and anaemias may only be diagnosed from such direct examination. Wherever possible, the results of a full haematological examination produced by a suitably experienced technician or veterinary surgeon, i.e. one who has knowledge of the species they are examining, should be obtained. This is especially important for the exotic species where the data with which the manufacturers programmed the machine in the first place may not be available or reliable.

Red blood cells

Morphology

Rabbit erythrocytes (RBCs) share the characteristics of typical mammalian cells, being anucleate biconcave discs. Their average diameter is 6.8 µm (midway between cat and dog) but there is a variable population of cell sizes between 5 and 8 µm. This wide range of cell size is reflected microscopically by the obvious anisocytosis which is seen on blood smear examination (Figure 3.1). This does not represent a regenerative anaemia and is normal for rabbit RBCs.

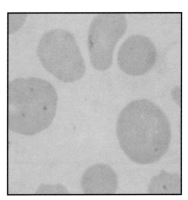

Figure 3.1: Rabbit red blood cells, showing normal anisocytosis and polychromasia. May–Grunwald–Giemsa stain. x1000 original magnification.

There may also be some polychromatic cells, schistocytes and stomatocytes. Reticulocytes are normally present at 2–5% of the RBC count (higher numbers are seen in immature individuals). It is also normal to find the occasional nucleated red blood cell (1 or 2 per 100 white blood cells) and cells showing Howell–Jolly bodies. Crenated erythrocytes, poikilocytes and red cell fragments are usually caused by poor smear preparation rather than disease.

Staining

If carrying out an in-house examination of a blood smear, most of the standard blood stains are satisfactory for use with rabbit blood and the choice is an individual one. The author's preferred stain is RapiDiff® (Cytocolor, Hinckley, Ohio, USA) as it is easy to use, economical and produces good staining of all the cells present.

Red cell parameters

- Packed cell volume (PCV)
- Haemoglobin concentration (Hb)
- Total RBC count
- Mean corpuscular haemoglobin concentration (MCHC)
- Mean corpuscular volume (MCV)
- Mean corpuscular haemoglobin (MCH).

The measurement of the various RBC parameters may be carried out manually by using a microhaematocrit centrifuge, haemoglobinometer and Neubauer haemocytometer. It is generally acknowledged that these methods may produce inaccurate results, especially if the technician is not experienced (as may occur in small practice laboratories or with species not encountered frequently). Submitting the sample to a commercial laboratory should ensure that reproducible and clinically valid results are obtained.

Clinical significance: These parameters are valuable indicators of disease. Changes in these values in rabbits are of parallel clinical significance to similar changes seen in dogs and cats and so may be interpreted in much the same way.

Thus, anaemias are divided into two types:

- Regenerative anaemia is characterized by the replacement of mature RBCs lost from the circulation by more juvenile forms. This may be seen as a result of traumatic blood loss, parasitism, haemolysis or lead poisoning
- Non-regenerative anaemia is usually caused by chronic illness, e.g. abscesses (large and chronic), pyometritis or hydrometritis, and tumours (the commonly encountered uterine adenocarcinoma of rabbits will also bleed readily so may produce a regenerative anaemia as well as a non-regenerative one).

White blood cells

Leucocytes (WBCs) display relative uniformity in appearance and function across most mammal species and this generality also applies to rabbits.

The description of the WBC component of a blood sample is made up of :

- Total WBC count
- Differential WBC count, expressed both as a percentage of each cell type present and also as the calculated absolute number of each cell type. This is calculated as [total white cell count] x [percentage of the cell type (expressed as a decimal)]
- Description of the cells seen.

Diurnal variations in some parameters do occur. For example, total WBC and lymphocyte numbers are lowest in the afternoon and evening, whilst neutrophil numbers peak during those times. Eosinophil levels increase in the afternoon and are at their lowest in the morning. Stressors (illness, handling, trauma) cause leucocytosis, neutrophilia and lymphopenia (probably due to an increase in endogenous steroid production).

Neutrophils (PMNs)

The average cell diameter is 10-15 µm and the outline is roughly round. The normal neutrophil nucleus is distinctly segmented and stains a deep purple blue; the segments are connected by thin strands of chromatin. The cytoplasm is clear and there are two distinct granules present; the smaller stain pink (and tend to give the cytoplasm an overall pink colour) whilst the large granules stain a deep pinkish red (Figure 3.2). The relative numbers of each granule vary from cell to cell and thus individual neutrophils may show differences in cytoplasm colour and granulation ranging from a deep red (many large granules) to pink (few large granules). This variable granulation has given rise to some differences in the classification of the cell (i.e. pseudoeosinophil, heterophil, amphophil or acidophil) but it is best to retain the description that compares it functionally with similar cells in other species rather than by staining characteristics.

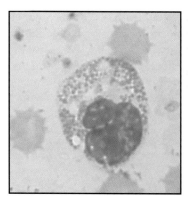

Figure 3.2: Rabbit neutrophil, showing granules. May–Grunwald–Giemsa stain. x1000 original magnification.

It is thought that bacterial infections in rabbits may be expressed as a neutrophilia and lymphopenia without an absolute leucocytosis. However, the normal values for different ages, sexes, breeds and husbandry may modify that impression and a lymphocyte to neutrophil ratio may be more valuable (if such data are available). Band forms do not tend to increase in animals suffering from bacterial infections, so the lack of a 'left shift' should not preclude the presence of such diseases. Steroids (endogenous and/or exogenous) will produce a leucocytosis and a neutrophilia, but these increases are not usually marked and an inflammatory response may be present and clinically significant without the animal showing a neutrophilia.

Lymphocytes

The average cell diameter is 7-10 µm for the small lymphocytes (SLs) and 10-15 µm for the less commonly seen large lymphocyte (LLs). Lymphocytes are normally round cells with a round to oval deeply purple-blue staining nucleus (Figure 3.3), which may have a slight indentation at one pole. The cytoplasm of the SL is sparse and may not appear to be present at all in some cells. The LL has a more abundant cytoplasm, which stains a mid- to deep-blue colour. Some LLs exhibit a perinuclear halo and there may also be a few azurophilic cytolasmic granules present.

Bacterial infections and the effects of steroids (endogenous and/or exogenous) may produce a lymphopenia but the overall WBC count may remain within the normal range if a neutrophilia is also present.

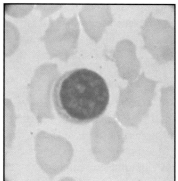

Figure 3.3: Rabbit lymphocyte. May–Grunwald–Giemsa stain. x1000 original magnification.

Monocytes

These are the largest nucleated cells in the circulation with a diameter of 15–18 μm. The nucleus is usually lobulated but may be horseshoe- or bean-shaped and has a lacey or stringy chromatin pattern that stains a purple-blue. The cytoplasm is abundant and stains a blue-grey mottled colour (Figure 3.4). Vacuoles are generally present but are not usually numerous.

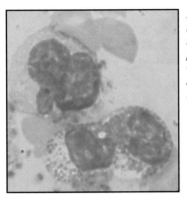

Figure 3.4: Rabbit monocyte with two neutrophils and platelets. May–Grunwald–Giemsa stain. x1000 original magnification.

Eosinophils

Cell diameter is 10–16 μm and the nucleus is deeply purple-blue staining and bilobed or horseshoe-shaped. The cytoplasm is completely filled with large granules, exhibiting a foamy dull pinky-orange staining (Figure 3.5). The granules tend to obscure the nucleus and this fact, coupled with the larger granule size, differentiates the eosinophil from the neutrophil. Increased steroid levels will cause an eosinopenia.

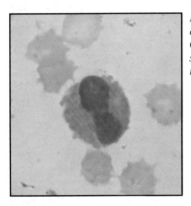

Figure 3.5: Rabbit eosinophil. May–Grunwald–Giemsa stain. x1000 original magnification.

Basophils

Cell diameter is 8- to 12 μm. The nucleus has either a band or segmented structure but is usually completely obscured by the large purple-black granules that fill the pale blue-grey cytoplasm. As with basophils in other species, their function in rabbits has not been fully determined.

Platelets

These are anucleated cell fragments 1–3 μm in diameter (although larger forms may be observed). They are round and have a pale blue cytoplasm (see Figure 3.4) containing reddish violet granules; clumping may be evident.

BIOCHEMICAL EVALUATIONS

Samples and sample handling

Either plasma or serum may be used for most biochemical assays but it is best to check with the laboratory or against the assay data sheet (if using an in-house analyser) for the preferred sample for each test.

Sample tubes (volumes 0.4–5 ml) for use are:

- Plain (serum), white top
- With heparin, orange top.

Heparin does not affect biochemistry values if it is present at non-optimal concentrations; 2 ml of blood may be placed in a 5 ml heparinized tube and accurate results will still obtained. Heparin is degraded in blood and this will allow samples to haemolyse and clot if there is a significant delay (more that 2 days) between sampling and analysis. It is therefore desirable to separate the cells from the plasma by centrifugation and submit (or analyse) the plasma as soon after collection as possible. Serum gel tubes allow the original tube to be used without decanting as the gel acts (after centrifugation) as a physical barrier between cells and serum.

Haemolysis is an undesirable artefact caused by poor blood sampling technique, overlong storage or disease. It will reduce RBC numbers and amylase concentration and increase levels of AST, ALT, LDH, CK, TP and potassium. Some automated biochemistry analysers may be programmed to compensate for this effect if it is not too severe but values obtained from haemolysed samples should always be viewed with suspicion and a repeat sample obtained.

Stressors such as in illness or due to handling (struggling) at the time of examination or blood sampling may modify some parameters; for example, glucose levels may be increased.

Aspartate aminotransferase (AST)

AST has a short half-life (5 hours) and is not very tissue-specific (having the same activity in heart as in liver, for example). This, coupled with the fact that AST levels increase after restraint, probably reduces its value as an indicator of any specific tissue damage.

Creatine phosphokinase (CPK)

Also known as creatine kinase (CK), the levels of this enzyme increase after restraint (as one would expect for a muscle-specific enzyme). It is useful as an indicator of specific muscle tissue damage.

Lactate dehydrogenase (LDH)

LDH levels rise after restraint and thus may not be specific for liver damage in the rabbit. If included in a biochemical 'profile', however, LDH level may be valuable when taken in context.

Alanine aminotransferase (ALT)
ALT concentrations show no measurable increase due to restraint and this fact support its use as an indicator of hepatocyte damage, in line with other mammal species.

Alkaline phosphatase (AP or ALP)
The rabbit is unusual in producing two discrete and individual alkaline phosphatase isoenzymes which show no obvious increases as a result of restraint and are thus thought to be good indicators of more chronic liver damage such as cirrhosis and obstructive disorders that cause biliary stasis.

Amylase
Amylase is only produced by the pancreas in rabbits, so elevated concentrations are seen in pancreatitis and abdominal traumas (including peritonitis and other similar abdominal insults). The enzyme is excreted in significant amounts by the kidneys (as well as by the liver) so raised levels may also be seen in renal failure due to reduced clearance rates. Plasma concentrations are also known to be increased by elevated corticosteroids (stress-induced endogenous increase or introduced therapeutically).

Lipase
The role of lipase in assessing clinical pancreatic disease in rabbits has not been studied but there is no reason to doubt that it is produced specifically by this organ and that significantly elevated plasma concentrations indicate pancreatic cell damage. It is likely that corticosteroids will increase serum lipase levels in line with the effect of these compounds seen in other species.

Bile pigments
A number of bile pigments are produced during the breakdown of the haem molecule by hepatocytes and are actively excreted via the biliary tree. Biliverdin is the primary haem breakdown product in the rabbit but this species also produces significant levels of bilirubin and measurement of this metabolite is useful in the assessment of both hepatocyte and biliary tree function. Bilirubininaemia is not commonly observed in rabbits but when present is usually the result of physical obstruction of bile drainage, e.g. by an abdominal mass or liver tumour.

Bromosulphthalein (BSP) retention testing has been carried out in healthy rabbits. Doses of 30, 60 and 120 mg/kg i.v. produced plasma levels in normal animals of 1, 2 and 20 mg/dl at 32 minutes post-injection. The overall rate of pigment removal is reported to be 1.8 mg/min/kg. A loss of more than 55% of functional mass is thought to be required before decreased clearance rates are expected. As in the dog, dehydration, shock and drugs that bind to albumin may produce falsely decreased BSP clearance rates. Other obvious causes of biliary obstruction should be excluded from the differential list before carrying out this test as they may lead to grossly decreased BSP clearance rates which may not be associated with hepatic cirrhosis or other organ-specific causes of bile stasis.

Urea
Urea is produced by the liver during the catabolism of protein molecules. This production is not constant but is influenced by dietary protein values, hepatocellular function, state of hydration, concurrent illness and other factors. The excretion of the metabolite via the kidneys is also not carried out at a constant rate. This casts doubt on the reliability of using the measurement of urea levels alone to assess renal function; other protein catabolytes such as creatinine are better used in this respect.

Urea may be measured in whole blood (often incorrectly known as blood urea nitrogen or BUN) or in plasma or serum. BUN refers to an outdated unit of measurement and should not be used.

Creatinine
Creatinine is a protein breakdown product that is produced in muscle at a constant rate and subsequently excreted by glomerular filtration at a similarly constant rate. The measurement of blood creatinine levels gives a good indication of renal function (a loss of more than 75% of functioning nephrons will reliably cause a measurable increase in blood creatinine concentration) but will not distinguish between pre-renal, renal or post-renal failures. Measuring both urea and creatinine is likely to reveal more information regarding renal function than measuring either alone. As both are usually included in laboratory kidney 'profiles', they are best assessed together to obtain a firm indication of renal function.

Urine specific gravity (SG)
Urine SG should also be measured routinely when renal disease is suspected. In pre-renal failure there is an increase in urea and creatinine (azotaemia) with increased urine SG. In primary renal failure there is azotaemia but urine SG is normal or decreased. Post-renal failure due to obstructive bladder disease is not uncommon in rabbits, due to their urine composition and subsequent urinary and renal calculus formation, and so must be included in the differential list of causes of azotaemia (see Chapter 6).

Phosphate
Phosphate (PO_4^{2-}) is excreted by the glomeruli and reabsorbed in the renal tubules so may be affected by renal disease. Any animal showing increased phosphate levels should be checked for renal disease, although dietary changes (including excessive amounts of mineral supplements and vitamin D administered by owners), intestinal disorders and haemolysis (more frequently a blood collection artefact rather than intravascular haemolysis) will also produce a hyperphosphataemia.

Calcium (Ca^{2+})

Calcium levels may be raised in rabbit blood (12–16 mg/dl) if the animals are fed high levels of supplements such as alfalfa (lucerne) and this may predispose to urolithiasis (even if this is only seen as a thick sludge-like urine). Management of urolithiasis may be made more successful if serum calcium is monitored too. Renal disease may also affect calcium levels but both hypo- and hypercalcaemia are common.

Potassium (K^{+})

Potassium levels are important in any species but abnormal findings are uncommon in rabbits. This does not mean that they should be ignored and both hyper- and hypokalaemia must be corrected as soon as observed. The same therapeutic guidelines should be used as for the dog and cat.

Glucose

Blood glucose concentrations may be modified as a result of disease or as a physiological response to stressors. Hypoglycaemia is usually seen in debilitated or anorexic animals. Hyperglycaemia is seen both as a response to handling (including blood sampling) and in diabetes mellitus. Diabetes is a relatively common endocrine disorder in rabbits and is expressed clinically as: polydypsia and polyuria; a persistently raised blood glucose level (>150–250 mg/dl); persistent glycosuria (confirmed most reliably by an owner carrying out testing with commercial dipsticks to minimize stress-related effects); serum potassium concentrations ≤ 1.0; and raised levels of triglycerides and glycosylated haemoglobin. As other factors can raise blood glucose (which may subsequently exceed the renal threshold and cause a glycosuria), diabetes mellitus should not be diagnosed on single test results alone.

Proteins

The albumin and globulin fractions of plasma are measured routinely and have the same significance in rabbits as in other mammals. At birth both albumin and globulin levels are low, but globulin levels increase rapidly as colostrum is ingested. Towards maturity both proteins steadily reach their normal adult values; globulins continue to increase but there is a slight reduction in albumin as old age is reached.

During pregnancy there is a decrease in total protein (TP) due to a decrease in albumin and despite a slight increase in globulin. Alpha-globulins rise sharply at the end of pregnancy and this increases TP. Albumin then decreases during lactation, with a lowering of TP. Sex hormones have an anabolic effect and increase TP, while thyroid and adrenocortical hormones have an opposite, catabolic effect.

Corticosteroid hormones

Corticosterone is the predominant adrenocortical hormone secreted in rabbits (the corticosterone:cortisol ratio is approximately 20:1). There is limited information regarding normal circulating concentrations and it is likely that, as in other species, these may be markedly affected by breed, husbandry conditions, sampling and analytical techniques, and other variables.

REFERENCE RANGES

There are a number of sources which cite 'normal' values for rabbit haematology and biochemical parameters but there is also a great deal of variation in the values from different sources. Much of the baseline data have been derived from laboratory animals kept in controlled conditions and may therefore be less applicable to the pet animal presented to the veterinary surgeon. Variation in 'normal' values will occur because of different husbandry conditions (house or garden rabbits) and interbreeding (for show purposes or as a result of indiscriminate breeding in gardens or for retail), as well as across individual breeds (dwarf to giant lops) and between individuals of different age, sex and metabolic activity.

The data in Figure 3.6 are derived from a number of published sources and represent the average and range of the values that those sources have obtained and accepted as originating from 'normal' individuals. In most instances there is no information available indicating the influence of breed, sex, age or husbandry conditions involved and so the data must represent values obtained from the 'normal average rabbit'.

Parameter	Average	Range
Total WBC (x 10^9/l)	8.55 6	5–12 5.0–8.0
Neutrophils (x 10^9/l)		3–20 1.5–4.0
Neutrophils (%)	48	34–60 40–70
Band neutrophils (x 10^9/l)	0.2	0–0.2

Parameter	Average	Range
Lymphocytes (x 10^9/l)	5.4	2–20
Lymphocytes(%)	53 47	43–62 20–80
Monocytes (x 10^9/l)	0.41	0–1.8
Monocytes (%)	3	0–4
Eosinophils (x 10^9/l)	0.26	0–7.0 0–0.8

Figure 3.6: Haematology and biochemical values for the 'normal average rabbit'. This table gives an overview of the data published and should be treated as a guide rather than a definitive source of reference values. ▶

Parameter	Average	Range
Eosinophils (%)	1	0–2 0–5
Basophils (x 10⁹/l)		0–0.84
Basophils (%)	2.5	0–1 0–7
Haemoglobin (mg/dl)	12	10–17.5 12–15
PCV (%)	40 39	34–50 33–47
RBC (x 10⁶/mm³)	6	5–8 5.1–7.9
MCV (fl)	69	50–75 59–79
MCH (pg)	21	18–24 16–23
MCHC (%)	33	27–34 28–36
Reticulocytes (%)		0–3
Platelets (x 10³/mm³)	290	240–600
In vivo coagulation time (minutess)	4	2–8
Protein (g/l)	61	49–71 50–71
Albumin (g/l)	31	27–36 33–50
Globulin (g/l)	28	24–33 15–27
A/G ratio	1.09	0.7–1.89
Glucose (mmol/l)	7.5	6–8.9 4.2–8.3
Urea (mmol/l)	3	1.5–3.8 1.6–4.3
Creatinine (μmol/l)	88	53–124 70–150

Parameter	Average	Range
Total bilirubin (μmol/l)		4.3–12.8
Triglycerides (mmol/l)		1.4–1.76
Bile acids (μmol/l)	11.6	3–20
Cholesterol (mmol/l)	1.1	0.62–1.68 0.1–2.0
Sodium (mmol/l)		134–150 130–155
Chloride (mmol/l)		92–120
Bicarbonate (mmol/l)		16–32
Potassium (mmol/l)		3.3–5.7 3.5–5.6
Phosphate (mmol/l)		1.0–2.2
Calcium (mmol/l)	3.55	2.17–4.59 5.5–7.8
Magnesium (mmol/l)		0.8–1.2
Iron (μmol/l)		33–40
Aspartate aminotransferase (IU/l)	57 < 50	33–99 5–50
Alanine aminotransferase (IU/l)	124 < 50	55–260 5–50
Alkaline phosphatase (IU/l)	51	12–96 100–400
Lactate dehydrogenase (IU/l)	187	132–252 50–500
Creatine phosphokinase (IU/l)	263	140–372 50–250
Gamma GT (IU/l)		0–5
Cortisol (resting) (μg/dl)		1.0–2.04
Cortisol (30 mins after stimulation with ACTH 6μg/kg i.m.) (μg/dl)		12.0–27.8

Figure 3.6 continued: *Haematology and biochemical values for the 'normal average rabbit'. This table gives an overview of the data published and should be treated as a guide rather than a definitive source of reference values.*

It must also be noted that different laboratories may use different methodologies for some assays and so will publish their own normal reference ranges. With the above in mind it would be prudent to view all laboratory data as being an aid to diagnosis and to monitor both the diagnosis and progress of each case by repeating blood tests (especially those falling outside normal values) whenever possible. Most laboratories will carry out individual tests or basic profiles to allow costs to be optimized.

REFERENCES

Collins BR (1988) Common diseases and medical management of rodents and lagomorphs. In: *Contemporary Issues in Small Animal Practice, No. 9*, ed ER Jacobson and GV Kollias, pp. 261–316. Churchill Livingstone, Edinburgh

Fowler ME (ed.) (1986) *Zoo and Wild Animal Medicine, 2nd edition*. WB Saunders, Philadelphia

Fudge AM (ed.) (1999) *Laboratory Medicine: Avian and Exotic Pets*. WB Saunders, Philadelphia.

Harkness JE and Wagner JE (1989) *The Biology and Medicine of Rabbits and Rodents, 3rd edn*. Lea & Febiger, Philadelphia

Hillyer EV and Quesenbury KE (1997) *Ferrets, Rabbits and Rodents: Clinical Medicine and Surgery.* WB Saunders, Philadelphia

Hrapkiewicz, K, Medina L and Holmes DD (1998) *Clinical Medicine of Small Mammals and Primates; An Introduction, 2nd edition.* Manson Publishing, London

Kaneko JJ (1989) *Clinical Biochemistry of Domestic Animals.* Academic Press, New York

Okerman NB (1990) *Rabbits, A Compendium.* University of Sydney Press, Sydney.

Romich JA and Ayers L (1994) Husbandry of the Rabbit. Part 1. In *Exotic Animals; a Veterinary Handbook*, pp. 64–70. Veterinary Learning Systems, New Jersey

AUTHOR'S ACKNOWLEDGEMENT

The author would like to thank Professor JE Cooper FRCVS and Mr MG Hart, both of Greendale Laboratories, for their valuable assistance in preparing this chapter.

CHAPTER FOUR

Respiratory System and Disorders

Anna Meredith

INTRODUCTION

Respiratory disease is common in domestic rabbits. The major cause of respiratory disease is pasteurellosis, but many other causes exist. It is easy to assume that all rabbits showing signs of respiratory disease are suffering from pasteurellosis, but a thorough diagnostic work-up should always be carried out. In addition, other factors such as environmental conditions and stressors such as overcrowding, transportation and intercurrent disease, can play an important role in the development of respiratory disease.

CLINICAL INVESTIGATION OF RESPIRATORY DISEASE

Clinical examination
Rabbits suffering from respiratory disease can be severely compromised and great care must be taken to minimize stress when conducting a clinical examination. Rabbits are nose-breathers, and mouth-breathing is a very poor prognostic sign. If the rabbit is severely dyspnoeic, mouth-breathing or cyanotic on presentation, allow it to relax in a darkened cage, and administer oxygen before proceeding. Signs of upper respiratory tract disease include nasal or ocular discharge, sneezing and snoring. Signs of lower respiratory tract disease include anorexia, depression, dyspnoea and cyanosis.

The nares should be examined for presence of discharge. This may be absent due to the rabbit cleaning itself with its paws, so always examine the paws and medial aspects of the forelimb for matting of the fur (Figure 4.1). A deep nasal swab of the turbinates is indicated if there is a nasal discharge. Insert a small (no. 4) calcium alginate swab gently into the nares along the nasal septum at least 1cm, and preferably deeper. Swab both sides as infection can be unilateral.

The eyes should be examined for the presence of conjunctivitis and dacryocystitis. The signs of dacryocystitis are lacrimal overflow and the presence of a white discharge at the medial canthus of the eye (Figure 4.2). Pressure over the lacrimal sac at the medial canthus of the eye will often cause expulsion of a white discharge

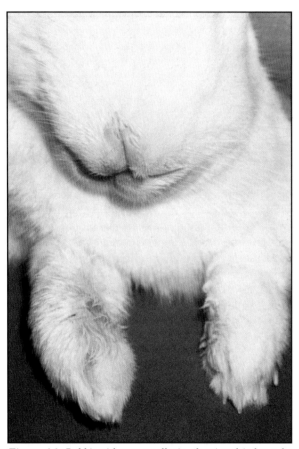

Figure 4.1: *Rabbit with pasteurellosis, showing dried nasal exudate on the medial forelimbs.*

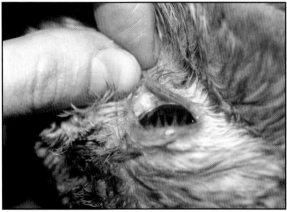

Figure 4.2: *Dacryocystitis: purulent exudate at the nasolacrimal punctum.*

from the nasolacrimal punctum (see Chapter 8). Flushing of the nasolacrimal ducts may expel a purulent discharge. Protrusion of the globe will indicate the presence of a retrobulbar mass (abscess or neoplasia).

The facial bones should be palpated and examined for lack of symmetry in order to detect any swellings, e.g. abscesses; the presence of facial paralysis should also be assessed.

The ears should be examined with an auroscope to check for signs of otitis media.

The respiratory pattern should be observed; this is more important than the rate. The normal respiratory rate is 30-60 breaths per minute, but this can vary widely depending on bodyweight and environmental conditions. A healthy stressed rabbit can have a very rapid respiratory rate, often exceeding 200 breaths per minute. Slow, deep respiration is abnormal. Note that nose-twitching is not directly associated with respiration, and cannot be used to assess respiratory rate. Breathing movements are largely diaphragmatic, and marked thoracic wall excursions are abnormal.

Auscultation of the thorax is difficult in the rabbit, as it is often hard to distinguish between upper and lower respiratory noise. A paediatric stethoscope head is useful. The lung fields are small in comparison to those of cats and dogs, and the heart is more cranially situated in the thorax. Auscultation should be performed over the trachea and sinuses to find out if abnormal sounds are loudest in these areas. Pulmonary râles and patchy loss of sounds can be detected with bronchopneumonia. Percussion of the thorax in larger rabbits can enable the detection of areas of reduced resonance due to neoplasia, abscessation or fluid accumulation.

Radiography

Sedation is preferable for radiography in the rabbit, but if the patient has severe respiratory compromise this may not be desirable, and a conscious dorsoventral view of the thorax may be all that is obtainable in the first instance. For the lateral view, draw the fore legs forward as far as possible to minimize superimposition of the cranial lung fields.

Interpretation of thoracic radiographs can be difficult. The pleural cavity is small and the heart lies cranially, close to the thoracic inlet. The cranial lung lobes are very small, resulting in a small retrosternal lucency, and there is often a lot of intrathoracic fat. These factors mean that it can be difficult to detect cranial thoracic masses and pulmonary disease, or they can, conversely, lead to over-diagnosis of these conditions.

Assessment of the lung parenchyma is complicated by the small lung volume, the presence of intrathoracic fat, and rapid shallow respiratory excursions resulting in difficulty in obtaining an inspiratory film. However, consolidative disease, parenchymal masses and the presence of a pleural effusion can be detected.

Enlargement of the cardiac silhouette is a non-specific sign of cardiac disease and should be investigated further using ultrasonography and ECG measurements.

In addition to radiography of the thorax, dorsoventral and lateral views of the nasal turbinates are useful. Increased opacity indicates the presence of exudate and decreased opacity indicates turbinate atrophy.

Ultrasonography

Ultrasonography is very useful in diagnosing pulmonary and pleural masses, and for guiding and directing needles when obtaining biopsies or aspirates. Cranial mediastinal masses can be imaged, but the position of the heart makes biopsy or aspiration very difficult.

Ultrasonography is also useful in the investigation of pleural effusion. However, it must be remembered that pleural fat can occur in strand-like structures that can be confused with fibrinous or granulomatous tissue.

BACTERIAL DISEASES OF THE RESPIRATORY SYSTEM

Pasteurellosis

Pasteurella multocida is a gram-negative bipolar coccobacillus (DiGiacomo *et al.*,1983; DiGiacomo *et al.*, 1987; DiGiacomo, 1989; Deeb *et al.*, 1990; Deeb, 1997). Many serotypes and strains exist, and the majority of serotypes isolated from rabbits are capsular type A, but type D isolates are considered more pathogenic than type A. The pathogenesis of *Pasteurella multocida* infection depends on the virulence of the strain and host resistance. In the 1920s, Webster and Smith published a series of papers establishing pasteurellosis as the primary cause of respiratory disease in domestic rabbits. They showed that rabbits challenged with *Pasteurella multocida* can do any of the following:

- Resist infection
- Spontaneously eliminate infection
- Become chronic carriers
- Develop acute rhinitis, pneumonia or bacteraemia
- Develop chronic disease.

Clinical manifestations of pasteurellosis are:

- Rhinitis ('snuffles') and turbinate atrophy
- Sinusitis
- Pleuritis
- Pneumonia (Figure 4.3)
- Pericarditis
- Otitis media or interna (Figure 4.4)
- Dacryocystitis
- Conjunctivitis

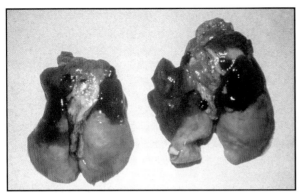

Figure 4.3: *Rabbit lungs affected with* Pasteurella multocida, *showing cranial lobe consolidation.*

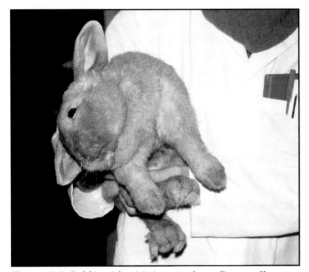

Figure 4.4: *Rabbit with otitis interna due to* Pasteurella multocida *infection.*

- Abscesses – subcutaneous, retrobulbar or of an organ
- Bacteraemia, causing acute generalized disease, pyrexia and death
- Genital infections (orchitis, pyometra) and mastitis.

Transmission is by aerosol, direct contact or fomites (DiGiacomo *et al.*, 1987). Transmission by contact occurs more readily from rabbits with acute rather than chronic infections (DiGiacomo *et al.*, 1987). Venereal transmission and infection of kits at birth can occur if genital infection is present.

The main route of entry into the rabbit is by nasal exposure or via wounds, and if colonization occurs, infection spreads to contiguous tissues or haematogenously. Many rabbits are subclinical carriers of *Pasteurella,* and the development of clinical disease is triggered by some stressor, such as high environmental ammonia levels, overcrowding, bullying, malnutrition, intercurrent disease, transportation or treatment with corticosteroids.

The role of the host immune response to *Pasteurella* infection is still unclear. Serum IgG to

P. multocida is not bactericidal and secretory IgA does not protect against nasal infection. Experimental vaccination can partially protect against severe disease but not against infection. The role of cell-mediated immunity is poorly understood.

Diagnosis

Diagnosis of pasteurellosis should not be made on clinical signs alone, although these may be highly suggestive. Direct culture of the organism and antibiotic sensitivity should be carried out wherever possible before the institution of antibiotic therapy (Langan and Schaeffer, 2000).

Nasal swabs should be inserted deep (1–4 cm) into the nasal cavity and obtained from both sides, as infection can be unilateral. Swabs from abscesses should be taken from the inner capsule wall, as the centre and any extruded pus is often sterile. *Pasteurella* can be difficult to isolate – swabs should preferably be inoculated immediately on to blood agar and incubated for at least 48 hours under aerobic or microaerophilic conditions. Colonies are convex and smooth, or may be mucoid, depending on the strain.

Haematology can reveal a heterophilia in acute infection, but more generally chronic disease is associated with a leucopenia.

Serology is available (ELISA) but is rarely carried out in general practice. It can be useful in detecting carriers or clinically inapparent infections. High antibody levels (IgG) correlate well with chronic infection. However, it should be remembered that it takes several weeks for antibody titres to rise, and antibodies in kits less than 8 weeks old are maternally derived. False negative (immunosuppression) and false positive (cross-reaction with other related bacteria) results are possible.

Treatment

Most strains of *P. multocida* are sensitive to enrofloxacin, trimethoprim–sulpha, tetracycline, chloramphenicol and gentamicin (Broome and Brooks,1991; Deeb, 1997; Mahler *et al.*, 1995). Antibiotic sensitivity should be carried out wherever possible before therapy is instituted. Great care should be taken when using gentamicin due to its nephrotoxic effects. Tilmicosin has been reported to be successful in treating pasteurellosis in experimental rabbits (McKay *et al.*, 1996), but is not generally recommended, as severe adverse effects, including anaphylaxis and death, have been reported.

Systemic antibiotic therapy should be given for at least 7–14 days, but prolonged courses (up to 3 months) are often necessary if chronic disease is present. Studies have shown (Mahler *et al.*, 1995) that although antibiotic therapy can control and eliminate clinical signs, it cannot eliminate the organism from the body.

Additional therapy includes:

- Oxygen
- Nebulization with mucolytics (bromhexine, *N*-acetyl-cysteine) or steam therapy to loosen and relieve nasal exudate if there is rhinitis or sinusitis
- Nebulization with antibiotics if there is rhinitis, sinusitis or pneumonia
- Nasolacrimal flushing
- Local antibiotic instillation for conjunctivitis and dacryocystitis (e.g. gentamicin, ciprofloxacin)
- Surgical removal of abscesses (see Chapter 13)
- Lancing, draining and flushing of abscesses
- Injection of gentamicin into capsule of abscesses
- Fluid therapy
- Assisted feeding if anorexic.

Control
Establishment of *Pasteurella*-free rabbits is possible by bacteriological and serological testing, followed by housing of negative animals together away from positive animals. Alternatively, Caesarean rederivation of the colony can eliminate the infection. There is also some evidence (Suckow *et al.*, 1996) that treating does with enrofloxacin during the periparturient period may interrupt the transmission of *P. multocida* from infected does to kits. Early weaning at 4–5 weeks is also useful.

However, such measures are often not practical for pet rabbits. Wherever possible, clinically affected and unaffected animals should be kept separately. The importance of good husbandry should also be emphasized – good ventilation, good sanitation and minimization of stressors. Sodium hypochlorite and benzalkonium chloride are effective against *P. multocida*.

No vaccine is currently effective or available for the control of pasteurellosis in rabbits.

Other bacterial agents causing respiratory disease
Bordetella bronchiseptica is commonly isolated from the nasal cavity of rabbits but is not associated with respiratory disease except under experimental conditions in young rabbits. It may, however, enhance colonization by *P. multocida*. It should also be noted that *B. bronchiseptica* is pathogenic to guinea-pigs, and these species should not be kept together.

Staphylococcus aureus and *Moraxella catarrhalis* can often be isolated from the nasal cavity and can cause disease if the mucosa is compromised (e.g. if there are high ammonia levels). *S. aureus* can also cause dacryocystitis, pneumonia and abscesses. Nasolacrimal flushing and fusidic acid eye drops can be of use in the treatment of *S. aureus*-associated dacryocystitis.

Mycobacterium bovis, *M. avium* and *Pseudomonas aeruginosa* can cause pneumonia and septicaemia in rabbits. *P. aeruginosa* can cause similar abscesses to *Pasteurella*.

Mycoplasma pulmonis has been isolated from rabbits with upper respiratory tract disease, but it is not clear whether it is a primary pathogen in rabbits.

Chlamydia can occasionally cause mild pneumonia in rabbits.

VIRAL DISEASES OF THE RESPIRATORY SYSTEM

Myxomatosis
The myxoma virus causes nasal and ocular discharge, as well as the more classical signs of oedema and skin swellings (see Chapter 9). Rabbits suffering from myxomatosis often develop secondary pasteurellosis.

Rabbit haemorrhagic disease (rabbit calicivirus disease)
Rabbit haemorrhagic disease, also referred to as rabbit calicivirus diseases (RCD) and viral haemorrhagic disease (VHD), emerged as a devastating infection of rabbits in the 1980s. It was first reported in China, and then outbreaks occurred throughout Europe and in Mexico. These outbreaks resulted in high mortality, and both domestic and wild rabbit populations have been infected. The disease recently spread to domestic rabbits in North America.

The virus is highly stable in the environment, but is inactivated by 1% sodium hydroxide or 0.4% formalin (DiGiacomo and Mare, 1994). Direct spread between rabbits, probably by the faecal–oral route, is of importance during an outbreak, but the virus can apparently be readily transmitted between populations by fomites such as food and water containers, and on the clothing of owners.

The clinical disease is acute, with high mortality (approaching 100%). The incubation period is 1–2 days, and the majority of adult rabbits (70–80%) develop disease. In many outbreaks, younger animals may be unaffected. In laboratory investigations of the pathogenicity of the virus, mortality was 95% for rabbits older than 9 weeks, and 50% for those aged 4–5 weeks. Animals under 3 weeks of age did not develop clinical signs of disease, but excreted virus and developed an antibody response.

Clinical signs
Rabbits often die acutely, with few clinical signs. Some may show a febrile response and become depressed, anorexic and lethargic, although because of the rapid progression of the disease, these vague clinical signs may not be noticed, and the first indication of an outbreak may be the death of some animals. Other clinical signs reported during outbreaks of the disease include tachypnoea, cyanosis, abdominal distension and constipation or diarrhoea. In the terminal stages of the disease, rabbits may have epistaxis and develop convulsions, or may simply become comatose and die.

Some animals recover, but it is not yet known whether the virus is always eliminated, or if a carrier state occurs.

Death is due to a coagulopathy, with disseminated haemorrhages in a wide range of organs. The degree of haemorrhage which can be seen at post-mortem examination varies considerably. Although the lungs are frequently affected, and may be very congested with obvious multiple haemorrhages visible on the surface, this is not a uniform finding.

The spleen and liver are often congested; the most consistent finding is a pale appearance to the liver, with an obvious reticular pattern on its surface.

Histopathological examination usually shows numerous necrotic areas in the liver, and often in the lungs, spleen and kidney, too. There may also be major thrombi in blood vessels, in addition to numerous microinfarcts. The thromboses in the pulmonary vessels result in the haemorrhage and frothy discharge in the nares and upper respiratory tract which is seen in some animals. Cerebral infarction or hypoxia may cause the neurological signs exhibited terminally by some rabbits.

Diagnosis
Diagnosis of the disease in an individual animal is based on gross post-mortem appearance, and confirmed by histological examination. When a rabbit colony is affected, the rapid progression and high morbidity and mortality seen are highly suggestive of the disease, even when gross post-mortem findings are not typical. Serological testing of animals that recover or that remain clinically normal can also be undertaken.

Treatment and control
Because of the rapid progression of the disease, treatment of affected animals has not been reported, and in any event is most unlikely to be successful. Efforts should therefore be directed at minimizing the risk of spread of the disease by effective disinfection of premises and isolation of any surviving animals, and protection of colonies and individual animals by vaccination. Commercially available vaccines appear to be safe and effective. After immunization, resistance develops in 1–2 weeks, but repeated immunization every 6–12 months (depending upon the vaccine used) is required to maintain protection. At present, it is recommended that vaccination to protect against VHD is not given concurrently with myxomatosis vaccines.

Since the virus survives well in the environment, all rabbits should be considered at risk, but those taken to shows are likely to be at greater risk of infection than other domestic rabbits. As with myxomatosis, outbreaks of the disease in the wild rabbit population can be followed by transmission to domestic rabbits, either directly or via fomites.

Other viruses
Herpes A virus has been isolated from rabbits with respiratory disease. However, the prevalence and sig-nificance of herpesvirus infections in the domestic rabbit population have not been established.

Coronavirus A, causing pleural effusion and cardiomyopathy, was reported in laboratory rabbits in Scandinavia in the 1960s. This disease has not been reported in domestic rabbits.

NEOPLASIA OF THE RESPIRATORY SYSTEM
Thymoma
The rabbit thymus persists into adulthood and thymomas of lymphoid and epithelial origin have been seen in young and adult rabbits (Vernau et al., 1995). Clinical signs include tachypnoea and dyspnoea, and bilateral exophthalmos has also been observed due to impeded venous return to the heart. No treatment is described.

Metastatic disease
Pulmonary metastases are common with uterine adenocarcinoma, and will also occur with other neoplasms (Figure 4.5). Thoracic radiographs should always be taken when undertaking surgical treatment of rabbits with uterine adenocarcinoma in order to assess the prognosis. Hypertrophic osteopathy has also been reported in a rabbit with a uterine adenocarcinoma-associated dorsal lung neoplasm (DeSanto, 1997).

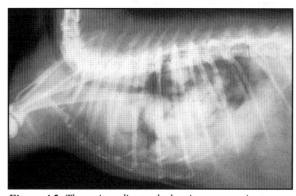
Figure 4.5: Thoracic radiograph showing metastatic pulmonary neoplasia in a rabbit.

Lymphosarcoma
Lymphosarcoma is most commonly seen in juvenile or young rabbits (Cloyd and Johnson, 1978). The pulmonary interstitium and mediastinal lymph nodes can be affected, as well as other visceral organs such as the liver, the spleen and the kidneys.

OTHER DISEASES OF THE RESPIRATORY SYSTEM
Respiratory irritation
High ammonia levels, cigarette smoke, dust and other chemicals can act as irritants to the respiratory mucosa and render it more susceptible to infection with bacterial pathogens such as *Pasteurella*.

Allergic rhinitis and bronchitis

Although information is largely anecdotal, exposure to allergens is believed to cause rhinitis and bronchitis in rabbits. A thorough diagnostic work-up to eliminate other causes of respiratory disease, especially *Pasteurella multocida*, must be carried out. If possible, the allergen should be identified and eliminated from the rabbit's environment. If this is not possible, antihistamines or corticosteroids can be used to control the symptoms; however, the use of corticosteroids is contraindicated in rabbits with chronic pasteurellosis.

Cardiovascular disease

Cardiovascular disease leading to pulmonary oedema will present as tachypnoea, dyspnoea, cyanosis or collapse. The incidence of cardiac disease in pet rabbits is unknown, but the author has seen several cases, including atrial and ventricular septal defects. Diagnosis and treatment is as for other species.

REFERENCES AND FURTHER READING

Broome RL and Brooks DL (1991) Efficacy of enrofloxacin in the treatment of respiratory pasteurellosis in rabbits. *Laboratory Animal Science* **41**, 572-576

Cloyd GG and Johnson GR (1978) Lymphosarcoma with lymphoblastic leukaemia in a New Zealand White rabbit. *Laboratory Animal Science* **28**, 66-69

Deeb BJ (1997) Respiratory disease and the *Pasteurella* complex. In: *Ferrets, Rabbits and Rodents; Clinical Medicine and Surgery*, ed. EV Hillyer and KE Quesenberry, pp. 189-201. WB Saunders, Philadelphia

Deeb BJ, DiGiacomo RF, Bernard BL and Silbernagel SM (1990) *Pasteurella multocida* and *Bordetella bronchiseptica* infections in rabbits. *Journal of Clinical Microbiology* **28**, 70-75

DeSanto J (1997) Hypertrophic osteopathy associated with an intrathoracic neoplasm in a rabbit. *Journal of the American Veterinary Medical Association* **210**, 1322-1323

DiGiacomo RF (1989) Atrophic rhinitis in New Zealand White rabbits infected with *Pasteurella multocida*. *American Journal of Veterinary Research* **50**, 1460-1465

DiGiacomo RF, Garlinghouse LE and Van Hoosier GL (1983) Natural history of infection with *Pasteurella multocida*. *Journal of the American Veterinary Medical Association* **183**, 1172-1175

DiGiacomo RF, Jones CD and Wathes CM (1987) Transmission of *Pasteurella multocida* in rabbits. *Laboratory Animal Science* **37** **(5)**, 621-623

DiGiacomo RF and Mare JC (1994) Viral diseases. In: *The Biology of the Laboratory Rabbit, 2nd edn*, ed. PJ Manning, DH Ringler and CE Newcomer, pp 171-204. Academic Press, New York

Langan GP and Schaeffer DO (2000) Rabbit microbiology and virology. In: *Laboratory Medicine: Avian and Exotic Pets,* ed. AM Fudge. pp. 325-333. WB Saunders, Philadelphia

McKay SG, Morck DW *et al.* (1996) Use of tilmicosin for treatment of pasteurellosis in rabbits. *American Journal of Veterinary Research,* **57,** 1180-1184

Mahler M, Stunkel S *et al.* (1995) Inefficacy of enrofloxacin in the elimination of *Pasteurella multocida* in rabbits. *Laboratory Animals* **29(2),** 192-199

Suckow MA, Martin BJ *et al.* (1996) Derivation of *Pasteurella multocida*-free rabbit litters by enrofloxacin treatment. *Veterinary Microbiology* **51 (1–2),** 161-168

Vernau KM, Grahn BH, Clarke-Scott HA and Sullivan N (1995) Thymoma in a geriatric rabbit with hypercalcaemia and periodic exophthalmos. *Journal of the American Veterinary Medical Association* **206,** 820-822

CHAPTER FIVE

Digestive System and Disorders

Barbara Deeb

INTRODUCTION

The rabbit gastrointestinal (GI) tract is exquisitely complicated (see Figure 2.4) and still only partially understood. Rabbits are 'hindgut fermenters', that is, dependent on flora in the large intestine to help break down fibre and provide nutrients; in this they share gastrointestinal physiological function with other herbivores like guinea-pigs and horses. In nature, rabbits are both grazers and browsers. They may select nutrient-rich leaves but are designed to obtain the most nutrition possible from fibre; fibre also drives gastrointestinal motility. Some nutrients are absorbed, while some are processed as caecotrophs, rich in vitamins and amino acids, and reingested (see Chapter 2). The rate of absorption and peristalsis depends on fibre intake. Thus, rabbits process grass and roots into the nutrients they need, and repay the earth with a rich nitrogenous waste.

Lapine efficiency of production makes rabbits attractive as prey animals. As such, they have evolved with behaviours which are in some way protective. They are social animals and form strong attachments. They are, also, acutely aware of changes in their surroundings and highly susceptible to stress, which has a major influence on gastrointestinal function. Stressors which may lead to gastrointestinal malfunction are:

- The imminence of a predation attempt
- The close proximity of a competitor
- The loss of a companion
- Destabilization of the hierarchical order
- A change in the living arrangements
- Environmental extremes to be endured.

Some rabbits seem to slip easily into shock when fear or pain is extreme.

Understanding the function and malfunction of the rabbit gastrointestinal tract has been problematical. Experimental studies of normal gastrointestinal function, flora, effects of nutritional variation, disease and its control have focused on laboratory rabbits or those bred for food. More recently, the popularity of rabbits as pets has shifted emphasis from herd health to diagnosis and treatment of disease in the individual pet. Herd health focuses on economically preventing and controlling enteritis in growing and breeding rabbits; while for pet rabbits, the challenge is longer-lived: extending the life of (mainly neutered) pet rabbits to up to 14 years. Veterinary clinicians and groups working with pet rabbits have contributed valuable and effective ideas, not only about nutrition and prevention, but also about diagnosis and treatment of gastrointestinal problems. In this chapter we will examine gastrointestinal problems and provide guidelines to differentiate and treat them in rabbits of varying ages.

For most rabbits, the first sign of a gastrointestinal problem is anorexia. It means 'something hurts', or food is not going through, or both. Peristalsis and appetite work together, each depending on the other.

ORAL PROBLEMS

Oral examination

Oral examination is difficult because the rabbit's mouth can only open to an angle of about 30 degrees, and the commissures of the mouth fold inwards, tending to hide the cheek teeth. Sometimes sedation or anaesthesia is required to perform a careful oral examination and treatment of cheek teeth. A nasal speculum or laryngoscope can be used to help visualize the cheek teeth. The tongue is manipulated using a gauze sponge. Magnification and illumination are very helpful. Radiographs aid in determining the extent of disease. Lysis around tooth roots and osteomyelitis can thus be observed (Figure 5.1). Further details of dental examination and treatment are given in Chapter 13.

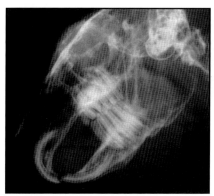

Figure 5.1: Radiograph of the head of a Holland Lop rabbit with tooth root infection and mandibular osteomyelitis.

Oral papillomas

Small papillomas may be detected during routine oral examination of rabbits. The lesions are usually seen on the ventral surface of the tongue and are viral in origin. The papillomas may be multiple, but rarely exceed 5 mm in diameter and usually resolve spontaneously within a few weeks, although they may rarely persist for several months. Treatment is not normally necessary, and rabbits that recover from the condition are resistant to reinfection.

Dental problems

Dental problems are common in rabbits. The teeth are open-rooted and grow continuously. Healthy teeth depend on conformation, uniform use and health of the periodontal tissues. Malocclusion may occur due to traumatic, inherited or infectious causes. Untreated malocclusion results in inability to eat, weight loss, malnutrition and death.

Incisor malocclusion

Malocclusion of incisors is easily recognized during physical examination, although often unnoticed by owners. The teeth grow long, eventually puncturing the tissues of the lips, nose, gingiva or palate. Treatment requires clipping and filing of overgrown teeth. The use of a drummel or dental burr helps to avoid tooth fractures (see Chapter 13).

Molar malocclusion

Cheek tooth malocclusions are more difficult to diagnose and treat. If tooth growth is uneven because of infection or uneven chewing, points or spurs develop on crowns, resulting in pain as they abrade the soft tissues. The rabbit favours the affected side, resulting in even more overgrowth. Some rabbits are very sensitive to pain and become anorexic when spurs first develop; others tolerate them until oral disease is severe. Eventually, spurs on cheek teeth may progress to extensions as long as a centimetre or more which cut into the cheek or tongue causing lacerations, ulcers or abscesses. One rabbit developed a spur about 2 cm long which extended into the pharynx and collected hair, resulting in severe respiratory râles and dyspnoea.

Tooth root infections are likely if the teeth appear discoloured, thickened or brittle. They usually lead to mandibular or maxillary abscesses and osteomyelitis. Cheek teeth should always be examined when swellings are detected in these bones. Epiphora is often a sign of tooth root infection, resulting from lacrimal duct blockage.

GASTRIC PROBLEMS

Rabbits are apparently unable to vomit because of the well developed sphincter of the cardia of the stomach. However, the author has carried out several post-mortem examinations of rabbits that appear to have regurgitated, resulting in aspiration of food material into the trachea and lungs. These rabbits were highly competitive for food, though not underfed. Healthy rabbits are eager eaters, but perhaps overeagerness should be discouraged.

In adult rabbits, the gastric pH is usually about 2. Bacterial infection is unlikely in this environment, but a variety of toxins can cause gastritis. Diet and ingestion of unusual materials must always be considered when gastrointestinal problems occur. However, the most common gastric problems in rabbits are chronic stasis due to accumulation of hair or foreign material, and acute bloat due to a foreign body or trichobezoar blockage. Gastric problems are more common during periods of shedding of fur and in rabbits with pruritus.

Chronic stasis

Signs of chronic stasis are decreased appetite and faecal production, and an enlarged dough-like stomach. Body temperature may be decreased or normal. The diet in these cases is often poor in fibre and high in carbohydrate, and the fluid intake is inadequate.

Acute bloat

Signs of acute bloat (tympany) may appear within a very short period: the rabbit seems fine, then suddenly becomes depressed, stops eating, drinking and defecating, sits with a hunched-up posture and may grind its teeth – signs of profound pain. Abdominal palpation reveals a large turgid stomach. The body temperature is usually subnormal; depression and weakness may progress rapidly.

Diagnosis

Radiographs will help differentiate stasis from bloat (Figures 5.2 and 5.3). Since the rabbit stomach is not normally empty, an extended emptying time of contrast material from the stomach is not a reliable indicator of stasis. The stomach is distended in both conditions, but contains considerably more gas with bloat. Although radiography is a useful diagnostic tool, it is a procedure that carries significant risk if sedation or anaesthesia is required, since many of these rabbits are on the verge of cardiovascular failure. Radiography carries risk in bloat, even without sedation or anaesthesia. It is therefore advisable to stabilize the animal with appropriate fluid therapy if sedation is likely to be required.

Blood samples should be taken for biochemistry and are useful for prognosis but, regardless of the results, treatment should be commenced immediately. A complete blood cell count is usually not informative.

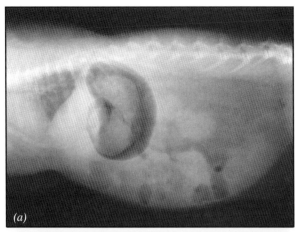

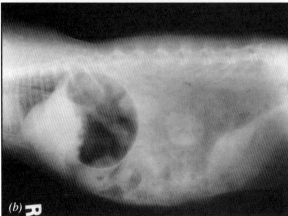

Figure 5.2: *(a) Air gastrogram of a New Zealand White rabbit with gastric stasis. (b) Air gastrogram of the same rabbit 2 weeks later: normal.*

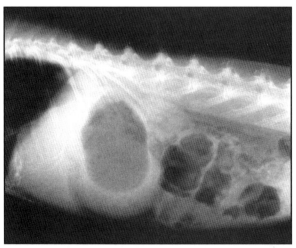

Figure 5.3: *Radiograph of New Zealand White rabbit with bloat; note gas and fluid in stomach.*

Post-mortem examinations on rabbits that have died from bloat or stasis have shown obstruction at the pylorus or in the duodenal flexure, with gastric or duodenal necrosis at the site of obstruction and gastric mucosal erosion and haemorrhage. Trichobezoars which have been found causing obstructions are usually not more than about 2 cm diameter and are truly rock-like (Figure 5.4).

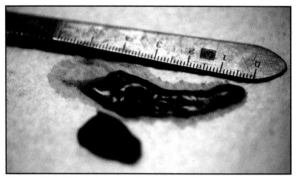

Figure 5.4: *Trichobezoar which caused intestinal obstruction, leading to the death of a Holland Lop rabbit; note necrosis of the duodenal mucosa.*

Treatment and prognosis

The prognosis for rabbits with chronic stasis is fair to good; for bloat it is poor to guarded. Surgery may be the only option in some cases, but it is hard to determine which animals would benefit from, and survive, surgical intervention.

Acute

The author has had some success in treating acute cases medically. An analgesic is given: flunixin, 0.5-2.0 mg/kg q 24 h i.m. or s.c.; butorphanol, 0.1-0.3 mg/kg q 4 h s.c.; or buprenorphine, 0.01-0.03 mg/kg q 12 h s.c. Warmed lactated Ringer's solution is given i.v. and s.c., and external heat is provided if the rabbit is hypothermic. Dexamethasone, 2-4 mg/kg i.v. or hydrocortisone sodium acetate, 10 mg/kg i.v., and enrofloxacin, 10 mg/kg s.c. are given. A plasma expander may be given intravenously.

If the rabbit is then stable enough, a stomach tube is passed for decompression from gas or fluid. Never decompress a distended stomach by needle puncture; the result will be peritonitis and death.

When improvement occurs, simethicone, 20-40 mg q 4-6 h orally is given, gentle abdominal massage provided, and mild exercise encouraged. A variety of foods are provided; interest in food is a good sign of improvement.

If improvement continues and gastric distension does not recur, metoclopramide, 0.5 mg/kg q 6-8 h s.c. is given. Enrofloxacin, 5 mg/kg q 12 h s.c. or orally, or trimethoprim-sulphamethoxazole, 15-30 mg/kg q 12 h orally; metoclopramide, s.c. or orally, and simethicone are continued until normal faeces are passed.

Chronic

The author's treatment for chronic stasis has been less dramatic. An analgesic is given if pain is detected. Warmed lactated Ringer's solution, metoclopramide and enrofloxacin are given s.c.; and simethicone is also given orally if gas is detected. These patients are usually discharged and continued on oral trimethoprim-sulphamethoxazole, metoclopramide and protein-digesting enzymes such as those found in pineapple or papaya.

Prevention

Prevention of gastric stasis and bloat includes careful dietary control: increased dietary fibre, reduced carbohydrate and the provision of protein-digesting enzymes during shedding. The owners should be advised to encourage their rabbit to exercise more and to prevent ingestion of undigestible materials, such as hair or carpet. Clients are also urged to help the rabbit remove loose hair during shedding and to control pruritus due to external parasites. However carefully the diet is controlled, with plenty of dietary fibre being given, an occasional rabbit may defy the best possible care and succumb to shock because of a blockage.

ENTERIC PROBLEMS

The 'enteritis complex', a term used for years in rabbit medicine, implies just how confusing and complicated enteric disease is in these animals.

Dysbiosis

Normal flora found in the rabbit intestine, especially the hindgut, are predominantly anaerobes: *Bacteroides* spp., Gram-negative non-sporulating bacilli, *Endosporus* spp., *Clostridium* spp., *Acuformis* spp. and Gram-positive spore-formers. Lactobacilli are not considered common normal flora for rabbits.

Dysbiosis refers to disruption of normal enteric flora, pH and peristalsis. This may occur as a result of stress, improper diet or administration of antibiotics such as amoxicillin, amoxicillin–clavulinic acid, cephalosporins, clindamycin, erythromycin, lincomycin and penicillin (see Chapter 11).

Mucoid enteritis

'Mucoid enteritis' is a term referring to a common syndrome of rabbits, usually of 7–14 weeks of age. The young rabbits develop enteritis and excessive production of enteric mucus, which may be passed in the faeces or accumulate in the intestine, causing impaction. A direct aetiology is not clear, although recent investigations have indicated that some animals with the constipative form of mucoid enteropathy have a dysautonomia, analagous to grass sickness in horses. The failure of peristalsis following destruction of the autonomic ganglia results in accumulation of material in the caecum, while the rectum and colon contain mainly mucus.

Bacterial enteritis

Bacteria associated with enteric disease in rabbits include *Escherichia coli*, *Clostridium spiroforme*, *C. perfringens* and *C. piliforme*. *Salmonella typhimurium*, *Pseudomonas aeruginosa* and *Campylobacter*-like species have also been implicated in outbreaks of diarrhoea.

Colibacillosis

This is caused by rabbit enteropathogenic *E. coli,* and occurs primarily in neonatal rabbits; it may cause 100% mortality. In post-weanling rabbits, morbidity and mortality depend on the serotype of the agent. Isolation of *E.coli* from faeces of ill rabbits implies association with disease. Confirmation of the diagnosis requires histopathologic observation of *E. coli* attachment to enterocytes. *Endotoxaemia*, systemic circulation of heat-stable toxin present in intact bacterial cells of Gram-negative outer membranes (lipopolysaccharides), causes capillary permeability due to tumour necrosis factor (TNF) release and sudden death.

Clostridial disease

Clostridium spiroforme is thought to be a major enteric pathogen in rabbits, causing disease and high mortality, especially in weanlings. Their susceptibility is probably because of their undeveloped normal caecal flora. In older rabbits, dysbiosis allows proliferation of *C. spiroforme*. The spores of clostridia may be endemic in rabbit colonies, and the organisms may be present in small numbers in the caecal flora of many rabbits. *C. spiroforme* produces an exotoxin (iota-toxin), which circulates in the blood stream and causes tissue necrosis thoughout the body. Such an *enterotoxaemia* may also develop from infection with other clostridia, such as *C. difficile* or *C. perfringens*. Rabbits affected by enterotoxaemia become anorexic, depressed, hypothermic, and pass watery faeces, or no faeces at all. A tentative diagnosis of disease due to *C. spiroforme* may be made by the demonstration of curved, coiled or spiral forms on Gram staining of a faecal smear, and post-mortem findings of necrotic liver, kidneys, heart, and haemorrhages in the caecal wall. Confirmation depends on demonstration of the iota-toxin in filtered supernatants of caecal fluid by toxin neutralization tests or enzyme-linked immunosorbant assay (ELISA).

Tyzzer's disease, caused by *C. piliforme*, an obligate intracellular, Gram-negative, spore-forming rod, may be endemic in many rabbit colonies. The disease takes a chronic form in older rabbits, but causes diarrhoea, depression and death in weanlings, especially when environmental conditions are stressful. The importance of Tyzzer's disease in pet rabbits is unknown. It is suspected when post-mortem examination reveals foci of degeneration of the heart and pinpoint foci of necrosis in the liver, as well as typhlitis and colitis. Confirmation of infection is made on histopathologic examination. Silver stains will reveal typical 'haystacks' of bacteria in the lesions.

Salmonella infection

Infection with *Salmonella* is rare in rabbits. When outbreaks do occur, the most common clinical sign is sudden death associated with septicaemia. However, some animals will show fever, anorexia and depression prior to death. Dyspnoea and cyanosis may also occur. Occasionally diarrhoea is seen, and abortion in pregnant females. Rabbits can also be subclinical carriers of *Salmonella* sp (DeLong and Manning, 1994). If treatment of an individual animal is contemplated, the zoonotic potential of this infection should be considered.

The source of infection in most reported outbreaks was thought to be contaminated feedstuffs. Confirmation of the diagnosis requires isolation and identification of the organism.

Yersiniosis (Pseudotuberculosis)
Yersinia pseudotuberculosis infection occurs in wild and feral domestic rabbits in Europe and the USA. The disease is usually acute, causing septicaemia and death, although diarrhoea occurs in prolonged cases. Pathological findings include microabscesses throughout the liver, spleen, mesentery and intestines, especially the appendix. Transmission is thought to be by ingestion of contaminated food. Zoonotic potential exists.

Viral enteritis
Rabbit rotavirus is probably endemic in most rabbit colonies, and weanling (3-10 week) rabbits are exposed, develop a mild enteritis, an antibody response, and then recover. The viral infection causes villous atrophy, affecting especially the ileum. Infection is likely to predispose rabbits to secondary bacterial infections of a more serious nature.

Coronavirus is also endemic in many rabbit colonies, affecting weanlings. Outbreaks of disease have included diarrhoea, abdominal distension and death. Testing for antibodies to coronavirus will demonstrate exposure. Confirmation of diagnosis depends on histopathologic demonstration of intestinal villous atrophy, crypt hypertrophy and virus particles in faecal contents.

Rabbit viral haemorrhagic disease (VHD), caused by a calicivirus, was first reported in Asia and Europe in the early1980s, then in Mexico in 1988. The virus is highly infectious and virulent, affecting rabbits 8 weeks or older. Morbidity is 70-80% of rabbits in an affected rabbit colony, within 2-3 days of viral entry. The course of the disease is rapid (7-14 days): fever, depression, anorexia, cyanosis, diarrhoea and death in most rabbits affected. Signs and pathology are associated with viraemia and acute disseminated coagulopathy. Enteritis is only a part of the total collapse of the affected rabbit. Epidemic viraemia, disseminated intravascular coagulopathy and venous thrombosis are suggestive of VHD.

Diagnosis depends on pathological findings and demonstration of the virus. A vaccine is available in Europe to prevent the disease. The severe nature of the disease must be kept in mind for all those working with rabbits (see Chapter 4).

Parasitic enteritis

Coccidiosis
Coccidians infecting the rabbit include *Eimeria irresidua, E. magna, E.media* and *E. perforans.* Eleven species of intestinal, caecal or colonic coccidia are documented (Owen, 1992), and have varying degrees of pathogenicity. With the exception of *E. magna*, which produces one of the largest oocysts (35 x 24 µm) and has a dark yellow-brown wall, and *E. media* (31 x 18 µm with a pink wall), the identification of species is difficult on examination of oocysts alone, and not practical. Unless the rabbit is compromised for other reasons, or the strain is pathogenic (*E. irresidua, E. magna*), coccidiosis is usually subclinical. Diagnosis of coccidiosis can be based on demonstration of oocysts in faecal flotations. Diagnosis of coccidiosis as a primary cause of enteritis depends on histopathologic demonstration of lesions and the ruling out of other causes. Coccidiosis is most commonly seen in young rabbits, as are enteritides in general.

Other protozoans
Other protozoal parasites: *Cryptosporidium parvum, Giardia duodenalis, Monocercomonas cuniculi, Retortamonas cuniculi* and *Entamoeba cunicula* have been found in the intestines of rabbits. There is no documentation that their presence is correlated with disease.

Helminths
A wide variety of helminths have been reported in wild and feral rabbits (Owen, 1992). *Passalurus ambiguus* (the common pinworm) is the most common helminth in domestic rabbits. The adult worms inhabit the caecum and colon, and reportedly are non-pathogenic. although the author has found occasional infested rabbits obsessed with overgrooming of the rectal area. The worms are passed in faeces; reinfection occurs by the ingestion of eggs. The worms can be seen in fresh faeces, or eggs seen microscopically in faecal floats or on sticky tape applied to the anal area and then examined microscopically.

Obeliscoides cuniculi, a trichostrongyle of the gastric mucosa, has been reported in feral rabbits.

In the Seattle area of the USA, a group of about 600 feral rabbits was collected and relocated to sanctuaries. Most were infected with coccidia, *Trichostrongylus calcaratus* and pinworms. They were effectively treated for coccidiosis with sulphaquinoxaline at 0.05% in the drinking water for 4 weeks and for the trichostrongyles with ivermectin, 0.2 mg/kg, repeated in 14 days, and for pinworms with oxibendazole, 15 mg/kg, repeated in 14 days.

Cestodes and trematodes have been reported in wild rabbits. *Cittotaenia variabilis* may be found in domestic rabbits allowed to graze on grass infested with the intermediate hosts, oribatid mites.

Treatment for parasites

Coccidiostats include sulphadimethoxine, 15–25 mg/kg orally q 12–24 h for 5–10 days, sulphamerazine 0.02% or sulphaquinoxaline 0.05% in the drinking water and trimethoprim-sulpha, 30 mg/kg orally q 12 h for 5–10 days. Benzimidazoles are effective in general against roundworms, as is ivermectin. Treatment of cestode and trematode parasites is praziquantel, 5 mg/kg.

Ileus and megacolon

Adynamic or paralytic ileus (bowel dilation or intestinal stasis), occurs due to impaired motor function, or is secondary to obstruction. A defect in innervation can be primary or secondary to gastroenteritis, peritonitis, toxaemia or trauma. Obstruction can occur due to a foreign body in the gastrointestinal tract, torsion, intussusception or neoplasia. Both ileus and typhlitis result in large amounts of gas in the intestine, especially the caecum (Figure 5.5).

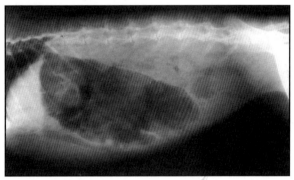

Figure 5.5: Radiograph of rabbit with typhlitis and ileus.

Megacolon occurs in rabbits and is typified by chronic accumulation of faeces in the colon, resulting in large clumps of faeces which cannot be passed easily (Figure 5.6). Although not documented, the condition is probably due to neurological impairment.

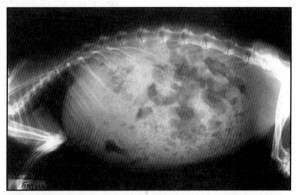

Figure 5.6: Radiograph of a rabbit with megacolon; note clumps of faeces in the colon.

Signs of enteric problems

Whatever the terminology or cause(s) of enteric disease in the rabbit, signs can be confusing, and often the cause is multiple. In weanling rabbits, the usual presentation is diarrhoea. In older rabbits, more frequently intestinal stasis or ileus occurs, and no faeces are passed. The rabbit may seem depressed or lethargic, depending on whether body temperature is abnormal. Physical examination and auscultation may reveal 'bubbly' and 'splashy' abdominal noises, indicating fluid and gas in the caecum.

Radiographs aid in diagnosis and prognosis. Faecal tests include: flotation to determine if parasites are involved; a faecal smear to determine if spiral forms of *C. spiroforme* are present; and a faecal culture to determine if an enteric bacterial pathogen may be present in excessive numbers. Serum chemistry and complete blood cell count results may help to determine the prognosis. However, treatment should proceed based on a tentative diagnosis only, if one is to save the life of a rabbit with endotoxaemia or enterotoxaemia.

Treatment of enteric problems

If the body temperature is below normal, the rabbit should be warmed using a heating pad, heat lamp or other means. Detection of gas in the intestine indicates the need to give simethicone, 20–40 mg q 4–6 h orally. Petroleum-based laxatives may help impacted matter or hair to pass through the intestine.

Lactobacillus spp. (probiotics) in powders, capsules, pastes or gels seem to be beneficial, although lactobacilli are not normal intestinal flora in rabbits. Lactobacilli can compete with pathogenic bacteria for mucosal attachment when dysbiosis and pH changes occur.

Caecotrophs from a healthy rabbit are the optimum way to reestablish normal flora. A slurry of caecotrophs with banana or baby food can be force-fed by syringe. If anorexia persists for more than a day, force-feeding is indicated, as hepatic lipidosis occurs rapidly in rabbits. Vegetable baby food, canned pumpkin or ground pellets mixed with saline can be used. A variety of foods should be offered: hay, grains, fresh vegetables and herbs; a sick rabbit often chooses unexpected foods when it starts eating again. Sometimes parsley, carrot top or hay can be introduced into the mouth and will continue on its way by habit. Exercise and gentle massage seem to ease colic and stimulate peristalsis.

Subcutaneous fluid therapy (lactated Ringer's solution) is almost always indicated for the anorexic, adypsic rabbit to ensure hydration and electrolyte balance: 5% dextrose is also given if the rabbit has been anorexic for more than a day. Intravenous fluids are advised if shock is impending. Analgesics are given to relieve colic: the author uses flunixin, 0.5–2 mg/kg s.c. q 24 h, or butorphanol, 0.1–0.5 mg/kg q 4 h s.c.

Cholestyramine (2 g/20 ml water orally once a day for 2 weeks) can be given to adsorb exotoxins if *Clostridium spiroforme* is suspected to be causing enteritis. Cholestyramine is a granular resin with affinity to hydrophobic compounds. It does not affect gastrointestinal motility and is not absorbed, but can dehydrate intestinal contents if not given with plenty of liquid.

The author administers antimicrobials in almost all cases of enteritis. Trimethoprim –sulphamethoxazole, 15–30 mg/kg orally q 12 h, or enrofloxacin, 5 mg/kg orally q12 h is prescribed for outpatient care. Enrofloxacin, 5–10 mg/kg s.c. q 12 h or chloramphenicol succinate, 50 mg/kg s.c. q 12 h is given in hospitalized cases. Unless gastrointestinal obstruction is demonstrated or diarrhoea is present, intestinal motility is stimulated using metoclopromide (0.5 mg/kg s.c. or orally q 6–8 h) when gastrointestinal stasis is suspected. Cisapride (0.5 mg/kg orally q 12–24 h) is administered if the rabbit has ileus or megacolon.

Prevention of enteric problems

Prevention of digestive disorders in rabbits hinges on understanding the rabbit way of life. A high fibre diet is essential to good health. Growth rates might be faster on high calorie feeds, but losses due to enteritis will be greater. Alfalfa hay should be fed to growing rabbits; grass hays to older rabbits. Most vegetables are well tolerated and appreciated by the majority of rabbits (see also Chapter 2). If a particular vegetable seems associated with loose faeces, its use should be discontinued. Rabbits cannot resist chewing on objects other than food: carpet, wires, walls, etc., and they sometimes are obsessive groomers of themselves or other rabbits. Therefore, one should provide safe, chewable alternatives such as plenty of hay, non-toxic twigs, untreated cardboard materials, etc. Rabbits are easily upset by changes in their environment, and stress increases the potential for digestive disorders. The following factors are all stressful for rabbits:

· The movement of a weanling away from its mother and siblings
· The loss of a companion (rabbit or human)
· The introduction of a new animal (a dog is a potential predator and a new rabbit is a potential competitor)
· Moving to a new home.

It should be suggested to clients that these changes be made as gradually and tolerably as possible.

It is important to know which agents may cause digestive disease in rabbits. Most are transmitted by the faecal–oral route or by fomites; thus, good hygiene is important. Most agents are inactivated by exposure to heat (80°F for 30 min) or 5% bleach (0.3% hypochlorite solution). A variety of other disinfecting agents are effective. Of course, disinfectants can be toxic, so they must be washed from contact surfaces. Rabbit colony caretakers must understand that sick rabbits should be cared for last, to avoid spread of infectious agents. However, for pet rabbits already sharing quarters, isolating a sick rabbit from a healthy one, which has already been exposed, would be detrimental to both. Daily examination of appetite and faeces of individual rabbits, careful observation of those showing change from normal, and veterinary examination and treatment of those with anorexia and diarrhoea or no faeces will help to avert loss due to gastrointestinal disease. There is no guaranteed formula for prevention. Even with the best care, some rabbits may experience enteritis.

HEPATIC PROBLEMS

Liver disease of rabbits includes hepatitis due to bacteraemia or viraemia, coccidiosis, lipidosis, toxaemia and necrosis, cholangitis, neoplasia and lobe torsion.

Coccidiosis

Hepatic coccidiosis, caused by *Eimeria stiedae*, is a serious problem in some rabbit colonies. Affected rabbits are thin, icteric, grow poorly and may have abdominal distension due to hepatomegaly and ascites (Figure 5.7). On post-mortem examination, irregular yellowish foci of necrosis of parasitized bile ducts are found (Figure 5.8). Wet mounts of liver foci or of those in the gall bladder will show all forms of the parasite. Oocysts are shed in faeces; sporozoites excyst in the duodenum; and merozoites invade bile duct epithelial cells, producing micro- and macrogametes, and thus oocysts. The prepatent period is 15–18 days. Treatment for liver coccidiosis is as for intestinal coccidiosis.

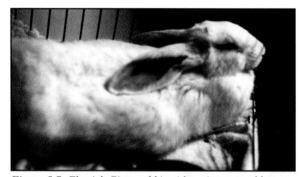

Figure 5.7: *Flemish Giant rabbit with ascites caused by* Eimeria stiedae *infection of the liver.*

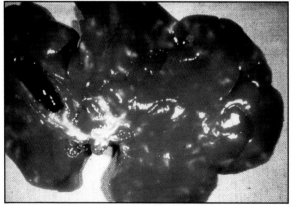

Figure 5.8: *Liver affected by* E. stiedae *infection.*

Hepatic lipidosis

Hepatic lipidosis develops rapidly in anorexic rabbits, especially if the rabbit has been overweight. For this reason, efforts must be made to ensure that there is positive energy balance by force feeding or injecting fluids containing 5% dextrose. Enterotoxaemia will result in hepatic necrosis. Early, aggressive treatment of enteritis is necessary to prevent this incurable complication.

Liver lobe torsion

The author has observed torsion (Figure 5.9) and ischaemia of the caudate lobe of the liver to be the cause of sudden death in several, otherwise healthy, rabbits. At least one of these had a history of extreme physical exertion shortly before dying. If the diagnosis can be confirmed sufficiently early, surgical removal of the affected lobe should be curative.

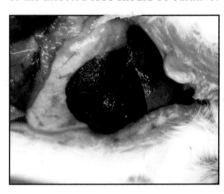

Figure 5.9: Torsion of the caudate lobe of the liver. The affected lobe is dark in comparison with the adjacent normal lobe.

Hepatic neoplasia

In addition to metastatic neoplasia in the liver, primary hepatocellular carcinoma occurs in older rabbits.

SUMMARY

Figure 5.10 shows the general diagnostic approach and treatment of rabbits that present with digestive problems.

REFERENCES AND FURTHER READING

Cheek PR (1987) *Rabbit Feeding and Nutrition.* Academic Press, Orlando.

Harkness JE and Wagner JE (1995) *The Biology and Medicine of Rabbits and Rodents, 4th edn.* Williams and Wilkins, Philadelphia.

Jenkins JR (1997) Gastrointestinal diseases. In: *Ferrets, Rabbits, and Rodents. Clinical Medicine and Surgery,* ed. EV Hillyer and KE Quesenberry, pp. 176-188. W.B. Saunders, Philadelphia.

Kraus AL, Weisbroth SH, Flatt, RE and Brewer N (1984) Biology and diseases of rabbits. In: *Laboratory Animal Medicine,* ed. JG Fox *et al.,* pp. 207-240. Academic Press, Orlando.

Manning PJ, Ringler DH, Newcomer CE, eds (1994): *The Biology of the Laboratory Rabbit, 2nd edn.* Academic Press, San Diego. Particular attention should be paid to the following sections:
- DeLong D and Manning PJ Bacterial diseases, pp. 131-170
- DiGiacomo RF and Mare DJ Viral diseases, pp. 171-204
- Hofing GL and Kraus AL Arthropod and helminth parasites, pp. 231-257
- Pakes SP and Gerrity LW Protozoal diseases, pp. 205-229

Owen DG (1992) Parasites of Laboratory Animals. Royal Society of Medicine Press, London

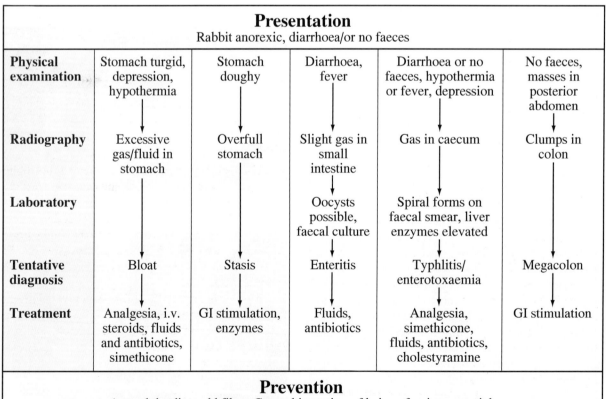

Presentation Rabbit anorexic, diarrhoea/or no faeces				
Physical examination	Stomach turgid, depression, hypothermia	Stomach doughy	Diarrhoea, fever	Diarrhoea or no faeces, hypothermia or fever, depression	No faeces, masses in posterior abdomen
Radiography	Excessive gas/fluid in stomach	Overfull stomach	Slight gas in small intestine	Gas in caecum	Clumps in colon
Laboratory			Oocysts possible, faecal culture	Spiral forms on faecal smear, liver enzymes elevated	
Tentative diagnosis	Bloat	Stasis	Enteritis	Typhlitis/ enterotoxaemia	Megacolon
Treatment	Analgesia, i.v. steroids, fluids and antibiotics, simethicone	GI stimulation, enzymes	Fluids, antibiotics	Analgesia, simethicone, fluids, antibiotics, cholestyramine	GI stimulation
Prevention Amend the diet; add fibre. Control ingestion of hair or foreign material. Hygiene in the rabbit colony.				

Figure 5.10: Diagnosis and treatment of digestive problems in rabbits.

CHAPTER SIX

Urogenital System and Disorders

Sharon Redrobe

ANATOMY AND PHYSIOLOGY

Kidneys

Rabbit kidneys are unipapillate. A single papilla and calyx enter the ureter which, in turn, empties into the bladder (Figure 6.1). In the doe the urethra empties into the ventral wall of the vagina. In Australia, rabbits

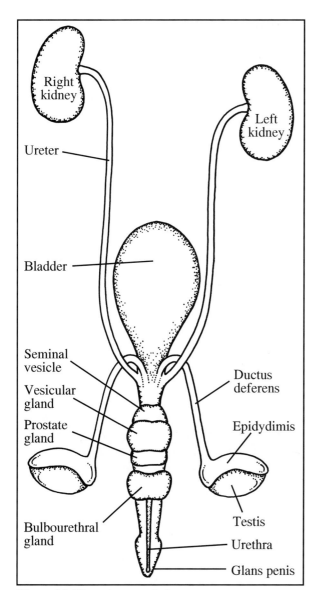

Figure 6.1: The male urogenital tract.

from the deserts or alpine zones have striking differences in their renal anatomy and physiology. The desert-dwelling rabbit has large kidneys with large medullas and can produce very concentrated urine. The alpine rabbits have smaller kidneys with a shorter renal medulla but larger adrenal glands producing higher levels of circulating aldosterone.

Urine

Normal rabbit urine can vary in appearance from clear through white, turbid, yellow, orange or brown, to red (Figure 6.2).

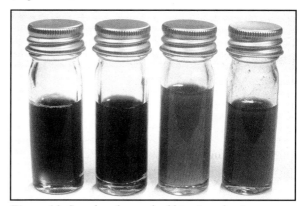

Figure 6.2: Samples of normal rabbit urine, showing variations in colour

The serum calcium level in rabbits is not tightly regulated as in other mammals and has a wide 'normal' range depending upon the dietary intake. Most of the dietary calcium is absorbed by the gut and the excess excreted via the urine. This leads to the production of a thick, creamy urine high in calcium carbonate. Excessive dietary calcium can lead to calcification of the aorta and kidneys.

The normal urine pH is 8.2 but this may decrease to 6.0 when the rabbit is anorexic or starved. Albumin and crystals of calcium carbonate and triple phosphate are commonly found in rabbit urine and are usually of no clinical significance.

Reproductive tract

The female reproductive tract (Figure 6.3) consists of two uterine horns leading to two cervices and a common vagina. There is no uterine body. The meso-

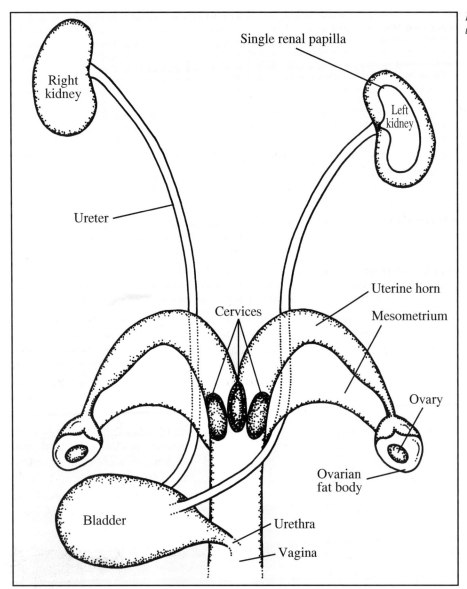

Figure 6.3: *The female urogenital tract.*

metrium is a major fat storage site in the rabbit. The female has four or five pairs of mammary glands.

The males do not have nipples. The male rabbit has two sparsely furred scrotal sacs situated cranial to the penis. There is no os penis. After the testes descend, at about 12 weeks of age, the inguinal canals remain open throughout life. Both sexes possess inguinal (or perineal) glands located just lateral to the vulva or penis.

URINARY TRACT DISORDERS

Red urine

As noted above, normal rabbit urine can vary in appearance. Red pigments may appear in the urine due to the ingestion of certain plants, foods, antibiotics or pine needles. Production of red urine may also occur without any change to the animal's diet and may occur in a single individual in a group of animals which are all receiving identical feed. This pigmentation is the commonest cause of red urine but haematuria can occur. This may be associated with blood from the genital tract (e.g. venous endometrial aneurysms, uterine adenocarcinoma, uterine polyps) or from the urinary tract (e.g. cystitis, urolithiasis, renal infarcts).

Differential diagnosis

- Plant material ingested leading to red coloration
- Blood in the urine from the reproductive tract (uterine adenocarcinoma, polyps, abortion, endometrial venous aneurysm, dystocia) or urinary tract (cystitis, bladder polyps, renal infarct, urolithiasis).

Diagnosis

Urinalysis must be performed to differentiate between blood in the urine and pigment. Microscopy may also be used to examine the urine sediment for red blood cells. Radiography and ultrasonography may be used to investigate lesions associated with the genital or urinary tract.

Treatment
No treatment is required for red pigmentation of the urine. This condition usually lasts for only 3 or 4 days and is of no clinical significance. Treatment for conditions associated with blood loss are discussed below under the relevant subject headings.

Urinary incontinence
Incontinence can be caused by spinal fractures, spinal dislocation, CNS lesions, CNS infections (e.g. *Encephalitozoon cuniculi*, *Toxoplasma*) or as a sequel to ovariohysterectomy. Incontinence must be differentiated from polyuria and from soiling of the perineal area due, for example, to obesity and lack of grooming.

Clinical signs
Clinical signs of urinary incontinence are urine scalding of the perineum, strong-smelling urine, dermatitis and ulceration of the perineal area.

Differential diagnosis
Other conditions that may present similarly to urinary incontinence include ectopic ureter, urinary tract infection, neoplasia and dermatitis secondary to urine scalding caused by obesity.

Diagnosis
A thorough neurological examination should be carried out to assess any neurological damage. Radiography of the spine and urogenital tract may be necessary to investigate fractures, dislocations and any underlying disease. Special radiographic techniques such as intravenous urography or myelography may be indicated. Laboratory investigations should include serology for *Encephalitozoon cuniculi* and *Toxoplasma* (see Chapter 3).

Treatment
The underlying cause must be addressed. Supportive treatment includes cleaning and drying of the perineum, including clipping away stained fur. Topical or parental treatment for dermatitis may be instigated. Some female rabbits are responsive to 0.5 mg diethylstilbestrol one or two times per week.

Urolithiasis/hypercalciuria/cystitis
Calculi may be found in the bladder, kidney, ureter, urethra or kidney. The formation of calculi may occur as a result of several factors, including diet, anatomy and (rarely) infection. Rabbits have an unusual calcium metabolism. Most mammals have a urinary fractional excretion rate of calcium of 2% whereas rabbits may have rates of 45–60%. The level of dietary calcium is directly related to the amount of calcium excreted into the urine. It is not unusual therefore to detect calcium carbonate crystals in rabbit urine. Uroliths are usually of calcium carbonate and readily visible on radiography.

Clinical signs
These include anorexia, depression, pain, urine staining, weight loss, anuria and dysuria.

Differential diagnosis

- Uterine adenocarcinoma
- Pyometra
- Hydrometra
- Endometrial venous aneurysm
- Dystocia
- Urinary tract neoplasia.

Diagnosis
A clinical examination may reveal a full firm bladder if urethral obstruction has occurred. Uroliths in the bladder can rarely be palpated. Enlarged kidneys may be detected if hydronephrosis has occurred secondary to obstruction. The rabbit may resent abdominal palpation or exhibit bruxism (teeth grinding) if pain is elicited on examination.

Plain radiography will usually reveal the discrete uroliths. It is common to detect calcium carbonate crystals or radiodense 'sand' in the bladder on radiography as an incidental finding (Figure 6.4). If the condition is clinically silent, no specific treatment may be required. Multiple renal cysts may be differentiated from hydronephrosis using ultrasonography.

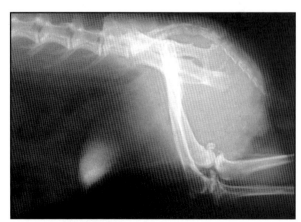

Figure 6.4: *Lateral radiograph of rabbit abdomen. Note the bladder 'sand' in this clinically normal rabbit.*

Urine is collected by cystocentesis, bladder catheterization or during spontaneous urination. Urinalysis should include measurement of pH and tests for the presence of protein, blood, crystals, casts and micro-organisms. Urinalysis will usually detect crystals but, as mentioned earlier, calcium carbonate crystals are a common finding and may be of no clinical significance. Ammonium phosphate and triple phosphate crystals may also be found. The diagnosis of crystalluria does not indicate urolithiasis; the latter must be diagnosed by radiography or ultrasonography. Proteinuria and haematuria may be associated with urolithiasis. Urine may be submitted for microbial culture.

Blood samples are sent for routine haematology and biochemistry to investigate the possibility of systemic disease and to assess renal function.

Treatment
Options for treatment depend upon the location and severity of the urolithiasis. Dietary modification is useful in managing mild cases and in the prevention of recurrence of the condition. A reduction in the dietary calcium level will lead to a direct reduction in the level of calcium in the urine.

The bladder may be flushed by introducing a catheter and instilling copious amounts of warm saline and suctioning the bladder contents. Most rabbits require sedation or a general anaesthetic to allow such manipulation. Inclusion of diazepam in the sedative or anaesthetic regimen can reduce the incidence of urethral spasm which otherwise is common following this procedure. The patient should be hospitalized until a urine sample has been produced to ensure that any urethral spasm has abated.

Cystotomy will enable removal of discrete uroliths or bladder lavage to remove 'sand'. Analysis of calculi and bladder wall culture may be performed.

Renal failure
Both acute and chronic renal disease, leading to clinical signs of renal failure, can occur in rabbits.

Clinical signs
Clinical signs of renal failure include lethargy, depression, anorexia, polyuria, polydipsia and perineal urine scalding.

Diagnosis
Elevations in serum creatinine, blood urea nitrogen and glucosuria are present in cases of moderate tubular damage. Serum calcium, phosphorus and potassium will also be elevated. In cases of chronic renal disease a non-regenerative anaemia may be seen.

Urinalysis will reveal isosthenuria, proteinuria, haematuria, pyuria and casts. Proteinuria is an early indicator of renal damage; this will occur before a change in the blood urea nitrogen is detected.

Urine culture should be used to check for infectious causes.

Treatment
Animals presented in renal failure should receive parental fluids, to promote an increased urine output, plus general supportive therapy. Antimicrobials may be needed to treat infectious disease, e.g. pyelonephritis.

Dietary changes include reducing vitamin D intake and calcium intake if required.

Prognosis
Recovery is possible with appropriate treatment in some cases of acute failure, but the prognosis is generally poor. Note that renal damage, which may be associated with mild/moderate proteinuria is common in rabbits infected with *Encephalitozoon cuniculi* (see below) and the renal lesions caused by this organism may be of little clinical significance.

Renal cysts
Multiple small cysts are found in the renal tissue of some rabbits. This is thought to be an inherited condition. Its main importance is as a differential diagnosis for hydronephrosis.

The condition is often clinically silent. An enlarged kidney may be palpated on clinical examination. Ultrasonography may be useful for detection and examination of the condition. There is no treatment. As the condition may be inherited (as an autosomal recessive trait; Lindsey and Fox, 1994), affected animals should not be used for breeding.

Urinary tract neoplasms
Spontaneous neoplasia may occur, e.g. embryonal nephroma, renal carcinoma, urinary bladder leiomyoma, and renal lymphosarcoma (usually associated with multiple organ involvement).

Clinical signs
The clinical signs vary according to the organ affected and the stage of disease. Signs indicative of cystitis or renal failure may be seen. The condition may be clinically silent prior to organ failure or detection of metastatic disease.

Differential diagnosis

- Uterine adenocarcinoma
- Pyometra
- Hydrometra
- Endometrial venous aneurysm
- Dystocia
- Urolithiasis.

Diagnosis
Radiography and ultrasonography of the abdomen are useful to eliminate other differential diagnoses. Biopsy (via exploratory laparotomy or ultrasound-guided percutaneous biopsy) of affected organs produces tissue for histological examination. Full body radiography is used to check for metastases.

Treatment
The neoplasm should be resected surgically if possible, e.g. unilateral nephrectomy, partial cystectomy.

REPRODUCTIVE TRACT DISORDERS

Endometrial polyps and hyperplasia

These tend to occur in intact female rabbits over 3 years of age. Endometrial polyps progress to cystic hyperplasia that then progresses to adenomatous hyperplasia and adenocarcinoma. Senile atrophy of the endometrium may also progress to adenocarcinoma.

Clinical signs

The clinical signs include intermittent haematuria, anaemia, decreased activity, palpation of a firm irregular uterus, and cystic mammary glands. The condition may remain undetected and may be an incidental finding at ovariohysterectomy.

Differential diagnosis

- Uterine adenocarcinoma
- Pyometra
- Hydrometra
- Endometrial venous aneurysm
- Dystocia
- Urolithiasis
- Urinary tract neoplasia.

Diagnosis

Methods used for diagnosis of endometrial polyps and hyperplasia are abdominal radiography and ultrasonography, and exploratory laparotomy.

Treatment

The treatment is ovariohysterectomy.

Uterine neoplasia

Spontaneous neoplasia may occur, e.g. uterine adenocarcinoma, uterine leiomyoma, sarcoma, vaginal squamous cell carcinoma. Uterine adenocarcinoma usually occurs in females over 2 years old. It is a common finding in older rabbits; some studies suggest an incidence of 80% in rabbits over 5 years. The incidence is particularly high in Dutch rabbits and moderately high in Californian and New Zealand breeds. Its occurrence does not seem to be related to the number of litters the doe has produced and it also occurs in animals which have not been used for breeding. Uterine adenocarcinoma is usually fatal within 24 months without treatment.

Clinical signs

The clinical signs include a bloody vaginal discharge, increased aggression, blood on urination, and cystic mammary glands. It should be noted that in breeding does, decreased fertility, e.g. reduced litter size, and increased incidence of still births and mismothering may precede the development of other clinical signs.

Differential diagnosis

- Pyometra
- Hydrometra
- Endometrial venous aneurysm
- Dystocia
- Urolithiasis
- Urinary tract neoplasia.

Diagnosis

Methods of diagnosis include abdominal palpation, radiography, biopsy of the uterus, and thoracic radiography to investigate metastases, which have a classic appearance of 'cannon balls'.

Treatment

Ovariohysterectomy is the treatment of choice to remove all affected tissue. Thoracic radiography should be conducted to investigate the possibility of metastases. Following surgery thoracic radiographs should be obtained every 6 months for the following 2 years to check for metastases. It is important to remove the entire uterus to prevent recurrence.

Pyometra/endometritis

This is a common problem in the rabbit. Common organisms isolated are *Pasteurella multocida* and *Staphylococcus aureus*. Less commonly isolated are *Chlamydia* spp, *Listeria monocytogenes*, *Moraxella bovis*, *Actinomyces pyogenes*, *Brucella melitensis* and *Salmonella* spp. This condition may be associated with recent mating or parturition.

Clinical signs

The signs are often non-specific, e.g. anorexia, lethargy, depression and weakness. Clinical examination may reveal an enlarged abdomen with an enlarged uterus. Care should be taken during abdominal palpation as the thin wall of the uterus is easily ruptured. Polydipsia and polyuria, with or without a vaginal discharge, may be noted. This condition can occur in virgin does. Chronic disease may present with no clinical signs although decreased reproductive output may be seen.

Differential diagnosis

- Uterine adenocarcinoma
- Hydrometra
- Endometrial venous aneurysm
- Dystocia.

Diagnosis

Pasteurella multocida abscesses in the uterus and ovaries have been associated with a mild normocytic normochromic anaemia, heterophilia, monocytosis and hypercholesterolaemia. Radiography may reveal an enlarged uterus. Ultrasonography may also be used to detect uterine masses. A Gram stain may be performed on the vaginal discharge.

Treatment
Mild cases may be treated with antibiotics and fluids. If an open endometritis is present, a guarded, deep vaginal swab may be taken for microbial culture and sensitivity. The animal should be thoroughly examined for abscesses elsewhere in the body. Ovariohysterectomy will resolve the problem. The animal should be stabilized prior to anaesthesia and surgery. Antibiosis and fluid therapy should be given as appropriate. The uterine contents should be submitted for microbial culture to permit correct selection of an antimicrobial therapy postoperatively.

Endometrial venous aneurysm
This is an uncommon cause of haematuria in rabbits. Blood from the vulva may be seen after or during urination. Abdominal palpation may reveal an enlarged uterus.

Differential diagnoses are uterine adenocarcinoma, pyometra, hydrometra, dystocia, urolithiasis, and urinary tract neoplasia. A mild regenerative anaemia may be noted. Haematuria and proteinuria can be seen. In rare cases the blood loss is life-threatening and therapy to stabilize the rabbit prior to emergency ovariohysterectomy is required.

Hydrometra
Spontaneous disease can occur, but is rare. Clinical signs are non-specific, e.g. lethargy and anorexia. An enlarged abdomen may be palpated on clinical examination. The condition may be clinically silent and detected on routine ovariohysterectomy.

Differential diagnoses are uterine adenocarcinoma, pyometra, endometrial venous aneurysm and dystocia. Diagnosis is by radiography, ultrasonography of the caudal abdomen and exploratory laparotomy. Treatment is ovariohysterectomy.

Dystocia
This condition is rare in the rabbit. The young are usually produced within 30 minutes although parturition may, uncommonly, take several hours. Obesity, nutrient deficiency, fetal deformities, fetal oversize, uterine inertia or a small pelvic canal (congenital or as a sequel to fractures) may contribute to dystocia. It may also be an early indicator of developing uterine adenocarcinoma (Weisbroth, 1994).

Clinical signs
The history should reveal contact with an entire male. The patient may present with anorexia, collapse, vaginal bleeding, straining, or a history of recent parturition.

Differential diagnosis

- Uterine adenocarcinoma
- Pyometra
- Hydrometra
- Endometrial venous aneurysm
- Dystocia
- Urolithiasis
- Urinary tract neoplasia.

Diagnosis
Abdominal palpation will reveal the presence of fetal masses. Radiography will allow investigation of the number and position of the fetus(es). Ultrasonography will allow differentiation between live and dead fetuses.

Treatment
The addition of extra lubrication per vagina and digital manipulation may extract the retained fetus(es). In cases of non-obstructive dystocia and where uterine inertia is suspected, 5–10 ml of calcium gluconate 10% followed 30 minutes later by oxytocin (1–2 IU i.m.) can stimulate uterine contractions. The doe should be placed in a dark, quiet area and left undisturbed for 40–60 minutes. If no young are produced, surgery is indicated once the animal is stabilized for anaesthesia. A caesarean section or ovariohysterectomy may be performed, depending upon the viability of the fetus(es) and uterus.

Pregnancy toxaemia
This condition is most usual during the final week of gestation but it can also be seen in non-pregnant or pseudopregnant animals. It is associated with obesity and recent fasting or anorexia.

Clinical signs
Pregnancy toxaemia is rarely recognized in the rabbit. Signs include depression, abortion and collapse. The rabbit may quickly progress to coma and death unless it receives treatment.

Differential diagnosis

- Uterine adenocarcinoma
- Pyometra
- Hydrometra
- Endometrial venous aneurysm
- Dystocia.

Diagnosis
Late gestation together with the clinical signs is indicative of the condition. Urinalysis will reveal ketonuria; acetone may be detected on the breath.

Treatment
Treatment is often unrewarding so the prognosis is poor. Fluid therapy, e.g. lactated saline and 5% glucose, and nutritional support is vital to redress the negative energy balance. Once stabilized, caesarean section or ovariohysterectomy is curative. Preventive measures include adequate nutrition of pregnant does and the avoidance of obesity.

Prolapsed vagina

This may be caused by straining due to urinary tract disease (e.g. cystitis, urolithiasis) or by a reproductive tract problem (e.g. polyps, dystocia).

Clinical signs

A mass with a lumen is seen protruding from the vagina.

Differential diagnosis

· Protruding vaginal polyp
· Rectal prolapse.

Diagnosis

Examination of the mass is required to determine viability and the extent of the prolapse. Inclusion of the urethra or bladder leads to a poorer prognosis due to the risk of urinary tract problems as a sequel. The underlying cause of the problem should be investigated.

Treatment

The prolapse should be cleansed and replaced if it is viable and shows minimal trauma. Retaining sutures may be placed temporarily. Amputation of the distal vagina or associated polyps may be indicated. The urethra should be identified and obstruction avoided.

Uterine torsion

This is associated with parturition. It may be related to poor handling technique of rabbit in late gestation. Clinical signs include collapse, depression, history of dystocia or imminent parturition. Radiography or ultrasonography of the caudal abdomen may suggest torsion. Treatment is by caesarean section and repositioning of the uterus or by ovariohysterectomy if the blood supply to the uterus is compromised.

Pseudopregnancy

This may follow an unsuccessful or infertile mating, but can also occur in group-housed female rabbits following a doe mounting, or being mounted by, another doe. Clinical signs are mammary gland enlargement and nest-making behaviour, which often involves fur-pulling from the abdomen. Diagnosis is made on the grounds of history and clinical signs. No treatment is required. The condition usually lasts 15–17 days and resolves spontaneously.

Cystic mastitis

This is a benign condition that generally affects intact does over 3 years of age. Cystic mammary glands may be blue but tend to be non-painful. A brown serosanguineous fluid may exude from the nipples. Diagnosis is by clinical signs plus examination of a biopsy sample or aspirate from the affected gland. The condition usually resolves with ovariohysterectomy.

Septic mastitis

Septic mastitis may occur in lactating does due to poor hygiene or trauma to the mammary gland. Pathogens include *Pasteurella* spp., *Staphylococcus* spp. and *Streptococcus* spp. Clinical signs include rejection of young, depression, anorexia, fever and lethargy. The affected mammary glands are inflamed. Diagnosis is by clinical signs, and examination of biopsy or aspiration samples from the affected glands. Aggressive antimicrobial therapy, fluid therapy and supportive care are given as required. The young should be weaned. Warm compresses should be applied to the glands three or four times a day.

Mammary neoplasia/dysplasia

Mammary neoplasia or cysts may occur in association with uterine hyperplasia/adenocarcinoma. The mammary glands are firm and swollen. This may progress to ulceration. Diagnosis is by histological examination of biopsy samples. Treatment is by surgical excision of affected glands or the affected line of glands. Ovariohysterectomy is recommended due to the association with uterine adenocarcinomatous changes.

Ovarian cysts/tumours

Spontaneous neoplasia may occur, e.g. ovarian haemangioma. Cysts are rare.

Clinical signs

Signs include enlargement of the abdomen, reproductive failure and change in libido. Alopecia may be associated with some types of ovarian disease. The condition may be clinically silent prior to organ failure, an incidental finding at ovariohysterectomy, or detection of metastatic disease.

Diagnosis

Diagnosis is by abdominal radiography and/or ultrasonography. Biopsy (via exploratory laparotomy or ultrasound-guided percutaneous biopsy) of the affected organ provides samples for histological examination. Care must be taken to avoid contamination of the abdomen with cyst fluid. Full body radiography is used to check for metastases.

Treatment

The treatment is ovariohysterectomy.

Testicular cysts/neoplasia

Spontaneous neoplasia may occur, e.g. testicular seminoma, testicular interstitial cell carcinoma. Cysts are rare.

Clinical signs

Clinical signs include enlargement of the testis, reproductive failure and change in libido. Alopecia may be associated with some types of testicular neoplasia. The condition may be clinically silent prior to organ failure or detection of metastatic disease.

Diagnosis
Diagnosis is by ultrasonography of the affected organ. Biopsy (via exploratory laparotomy or ultrasound-guided percutaneous biopsy) of the affected organ provides samples for histological examination. Full body radiography is used to check for metastases.

Treatment
Treatment is by castration.

Orchitis/epididymitis

This may occur in myxomatosis, pasteurellosis or other bacterial infections. Haematogenous spread of bacteria may occur or infection may arise from bites from other rabbits. The clinical signs are infertility and enlarged swollen testes. Differential diagnoses are neoplasia and epididymal cysts. Diagnosis is by ultrasonography of the affected organ and examination of biopsy material. Treatment is by antibiosis; castration may be required if the disease is severe or unresponsive to medical therapy.

INFECTIONS AFFECTING THE UROGENITAL TRACT

Encephalitozoon cuniculi

Encephalitozoon cuniculi is a protozoan that infects the brain and kidneys. It is transmitted via the urine of infected rabbits.

Clinical signs
The infection may be latent and cause no clinical signs; however, some rabits may present with a variety of signs including those of kidney disease, muscle weakness (ataxia, paresis), emaciation, polyuria and polydipsia, neurological signs (torticollis, tremors, convulsions) and death.

Differential diagnosis

- Toxoplasmosis
- *Baylisascaris procyonis* infection
- Listeriosis
- Pasteurellosis.

Diagnosis
Antibody tests and examination of kidney biopsy specimens are useful. Antibodies can be detected in the blood 2 weeks before the organism is detected in the kidney. However, many rabbits have antibodies to the organism without showing clinical signs. Histological changes in the kidney are noted 5 weeks after the appearance of antibodies to the organism. Serological tests include immunofluorescence, complement fixation, microagglutination, Indian ink and microbead agglutination reactions. Intradermal skin testing and histology may also be used. The intradermal skin test has been shown to correlate best with detectable lesions

in affected rabbits. Chronic interstitial nephritis and tubular degeneration can be noted on histopathology of kidney samples.

Treatment
No effective treatment regime has been established. The use of either albendazole or oxfenbendazole has been reported to reduce clinical signs of the infection.

Myxomatosis

Myxomatosis is caused by a poxvirus that is spread by biting insects, typically the rabbit flea (see Chapter 9). This disease has been seen in house rabbits without access to outdoors and so all pet rabbits should be considered to be at risk.

Clinical signs
Oedema of the head, ears, eyelids and genitalia (Figure 6.5) is followed by diffuse oedematous swellings (pseudotumours). The disease is rapidly fatal in susceptible animals. Some animals may have a more chronic course of infection.

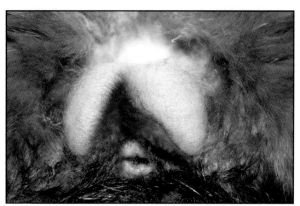

Figure 6.5: *Swollen testis associated with myxomatosis.*

Diagnosis
Diagnosis is by clinical signs and serology.

Treatment
There is no specific treatment available. Supportive care may be useful in those patients with some innate resistance to the disease; some animals may recover but the prognosis is poor. Prevention is by routine vaccination and vector control.

Rabbit syphilis

Treponema cuniculi is a spirochaete transmitted by genital contact. The disease affects the mucocutaneous junctions of the external genitalia, lips, face, eyes and nostrils. Autoinfection will spread the infection around the body. The infection is not zoonotic (see also Chapter 9).

Clinical signs
Minute vesicles develop into ulcerations and proliferative crusting at the mucocutaneous junctions, e.g.

nose, eyes, vulva, prepuce. Lesions may be seen on the forefeet where the animal has wiped the mucous membranes of the face. The rabbit is not generally systemically ill. This condition may be associated with infertility still-births and metritis.

Differential diagnosis

- Dermatophytosis
- Autoimmune disease.

Diagnosis

The clinical signs are highly suggestive of the condition. Deep skin scrapings may be submitted for dark field microscopy. Biopsy specimens of the lesions are stained with silver stain to reveal the organism. False negatives are common. Serological tests are available, including an ELISA test and a rapid plasma reagin test. Response to treatment can be dramatic and is used as a diagnostic tool.

Treatment

The organism is extremely sensitive to penicillin. One dose of penicillin at 50,000 IU by intramuscular injection at 7–10 day intervals can lead to resolution of clinical signs. The treatment may be repeated two or three times in severe infections. The rabbit should be observed for signs of dysbiosis (e.g. diarrhoea) caused by the treatment, although the single weekly dose method carries a very low risk.

REFERENCES AND FURTHER READING

Cox JC and Gallichio HA (1978) Serological and histological studies on adult rabbits with recent, naturally acquired encephalitozoonosis. *Research in Veterinary Science* **24**, 260–261

Hillyer EV (1994) Pet rabbits. *Veterinary Clinics of North America: Small Animal Practice* **24**, 25–66

Kimman TG and Akkermans JP (1987) *E. cuniculi* in a rabbit breeding colony. *Tijdscrift Diergeneeskunde* **112**, 1405–1409

Lindsey J.R and Fox RR (1994) Inherited diseases and variations. In *The Biology of the Laboratory Rabbit, 2nd edn,* ed. PJ Manning, DH Ringler and CE Newcomer, pp. 293–319. Academic Press, New York

Pakes SP, Shadduck JA, Feldman DB and Moore JA (1984) Comparison of tests for the diagnosis of spontaneous encephalitozoonosis in rabbits. *Laboratory Animal Science* **34**, 356–9

Paul-Murphy J and Ramer JC (1998) Urgent care of the pet rabbit. *Veterinary Clinics of North America: Exotic Animal Practice* **1**, 127–152

Weisbroth SH (1994) Neoplastic diseases. In *The Biology of the Laboratory Rabbit, 2nd edn,* ed. PJ Manning, DH Ringler and CE Newcomer, pp. 259–292. Academic Press, New York

Yamini B and Stein S (1989) Abortion, still birth, neonatal death and nutritional myodegeneration in a rabbit breeding colony. Journal of the American Veterinary Medical Association **194**, 561–562

CHAPTER SEVEN

Nervous System and Disorders

Pip Boydell

INTRODUCTION

The investigation of rabbits presented with neurological signs does not differ significantly from a neurological work-up in other companion animal species and should follow a similar pattern. An understanding of the functional organization of the nervous system is necessary for the diagnosis, prognosis and treatment of neurological problems. This chapter is not the place for a description of examination techniques and lesion localization; there are numerous veterinary texts that cover the basic neurological examination in some detail and many features can be extrapolated from those used in other species. Rather, this chapter will outline some of the common conditions that may present to the general practitioner.

Aetiologies for neurological disease include:

- Infection
- Trauma
- Neoplasia
- Poisoning
- Metabolic disorders
- Congenital/Inherited disorders.

The vast majority of presentations will be a result of infection or trauma.

POSTERIOR PARALYSIS AND PARESIS

Fractures of the lumbar vertebrae (Figure 7.1), particularly L7, are common in rabbits and are often associated with struggling during handling if the hindquarters are not supported adequately. The struggling rabbit can kick and twist to exert abnormal stresses on these vertebrae. This behaviour may also lead to dislocation of the spine in this region. The rabbit's spinal cord extends the length of the spinal column, unlike that in dogs, and any lower spinal injury will affect the upper motor neurones of the spinal cord itself, in addition to the lower motor neurones in that region. Depending on the site and severity of the injury, there may be interference with bladder control, anal function, hindlimb

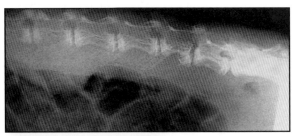

Figure 7.1: Lateral and dorsoventral radiographs of lumbar fractures.

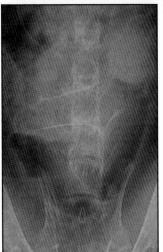

reflexes and sensation. At neurological examination the absence of deep pain sensation indicates a poor prognosis though this test is not always reliable in the rabbit, where signs of pain may be concealed and the behavioural response may be difficult to ascertain. A withdrawal reaction restricted to the hindlimbs might be a purely local reflex and does not confirm a functionally intact spinal cord. Radiography, including myelography if necessary (Figure 7.2), may confirm the site of the injury and the degree of displacement.

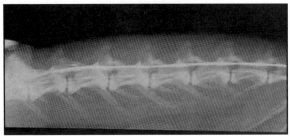

Figure 7.2: Normal myelogram.

If the spinal cord is transected, euthanasia might be considered, though some paraplegic house rabbits can continue a satisfactory lifestyle if the owners can devote sufficient attention to the prevention of problems associated with urinary retention, faecal and urinary incontinence and pressure sores. Some rabbits will tolerate the use of a trolley to support the hindquarters and will continue to lead a life of apparent good quality (Figure 7.3). Where there is some chance of return of neurological function similar care is necessary.

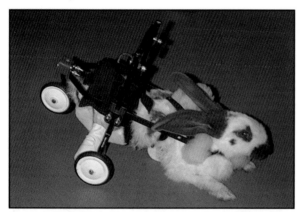

Figure 7.3: Rabbit with posterior paralysis in a cart.

In the acute presentation, the role of methylprednisolone remains unproven but many clinical neurologists would consider the administration of this agent. Reports of surgical intervention in such cases have not been published. If the spinal cord remains intact but the spine is unstable, then stabilization of the fracture/luxation might be performed (Figure 7.4). One predisposing factor is that many pet rabbits, particularly those housed in a small hutch with minimal opportunity to exercise, tend to have a fairly sedentary existence and the bone density may be poor. This increases the risk of fracture when inappropriate stresses are applied and can interfere with surgical fixation.

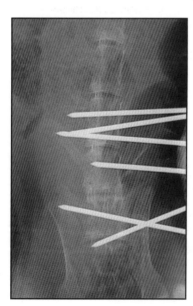

Figure 7.4: Fixation of lumbar fracture.

Disc disease is rare but has been reported. Nontraumatic spinal disease is uncommon, but congenital anomalies such as hemivertebrae (Figure 7.5a) and other anomalies (Figure 7.5b) may be seen occasionally; however, these may be asymptomatic. To the author's knowledge, spinal neoplasia has not been described in pet rabbits; however, this differential cannot be excluded absolutely. Meningitis associated with encephalitozoonosis or other infections may be considered, particularly if there is no evidence of trauma. Analysis of cerebrospinal fluid may show a pleocytosis in such cases but, in the author's experience, this examination is generally unrewarding.

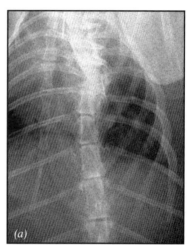
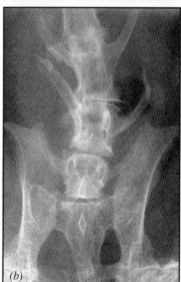

Figure 7.5:
(a) Hemivertebrae.
(b) Congenital defect of lumbar spine.

Splayleg

This is an inherited condition where young rabbits lose the ability to adduct the limbs. The disorder may affect all limbs, or primarily the fore- or hindlimbs. The condition may be relatively mild, allowing some clumsy movement, or so severe that the animal is completely paralysed. There may be skeletal deformity, particularly of the hindlimbs. The condition may be caused by a variety of different conditions, but all carry a poor prognosis. Although a few individuals recover some limb function, euthanasia is advisable for most affected animals. Since some of the causes of the condition are inherited, breeding from the animal's parents should be discouraged.

VESTIBULAR DISEASE

Possibly the commonest neurological presentation in pet rabbits is head tilt, a sign of vestibular disease. This may be accompanied by ataxia, falling or rolling and nystagmus. This syndrome may be divided into central or peripheral, which have different implications for therapy and prognosis. Peripheral vestibular disease usually results from otitis media/interna and is often associated with *Pasteurella multocida* infection. Central vestibular disease is more often associated with *Encephalitozoon cuniculi* infection (see Chapter 6) as a result of a granulomatous meningoencephalomyelitis. A positive blood titre provides circumstantial evidence, though many apparently normal rabbits will have significant titres and the test is better used to rule out the possibility of this disease if serology is negative. Demonstration of the organism by cytology is required for a definitive diagnosis. It has been suggested that dwarf breeds have a predisposition to encephalitozoonosis whereas standard breeds are more likely to suffer from otitis associated with pasteurellosis. This has implications in formulating a prognosis and establishing a treatment protocol.

Radiography, even computed tomography, of the tympanic bullae, may help to demonstrate otitis media, and flushing of the middle ear cavity can allow sampling for microbiological studies while removing exudate. Treatment with the appropriate antibiotic is indicated (see Chapter 11), though there may be minimal improvement seen; the incorporation of corticosteroids into the regime might be considered, but is controversial. The use of this symptomatic treatment as a last resort may reduce inflammation or secondary CNS oedema to allow continuation of an adequate lifestyle for some time. Anecdotally, some patients respond and do not relapse when the effects of steroid administration are expected to have diminished. However, one should always be aware of the potential for deleterious side effects associated with corticosteroids, and symptomatic treatment without demonstrated clinical justification should be reserved for those cases where other options are no longer available, or have been offered but declined by the owner. Use of bulla osteotomy as a treatment for middle ear disease associated with bacterial infection has been proposed (see Chapter 13). Brain scanning may also demonstrate a CNS lesion but confirmation of encephalitozoonosis still requires biopsy. Treatment with albendazole may be of some benefit in occasional cases, but many affected patients will not respond and euthanasia may be considered if the rabbit is unable to cope. Symptomatic treatment with antibiotics and, possibly, corticosteroids may allow a reasonable quality of life, but the possibility of spontaneous resolution cannot be excluded, though some neurological deficit often remains. *E. cuniculi* is the cause of a zoonosis and may be of concern to immunosuppressed people. 'Stargazing' (Figure 7.6) may be seen occasionally; this may be another feature of *E. cuniculi* infection. Similarly, herpes viral encephalitis has been reported in rabbits, both experimentally and following suspected infection from the owner.

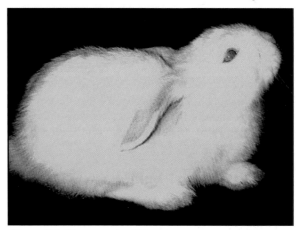

Figure 7.6: *'Stargazer' rabbit.*

SEIZURES

Epilepsy
Primary epilepsy has been described, but the majority of cases are thought to be associated with encephalitozoonosis or other forms of meningitis. Responsible organisms may include *Toxoplasma, Sarcocystis, Pasteurella*, and *Listeria*. Epileptiform fits may also result from hypoxia associated with pneumonia, empyema or anaesthetic accidents.

In general, the aetiology will not be confirmed and symptomatic treatment may be attempted with oral phenobarbitone elixir and antibiotic cover. Rectal diazepam may be given by the owner to treat occasional seizure episodes, or if cluster attacks occur.

Heat Stress
This can result from confinement in poorly ventilated accommodation or in direct sunlight during hot sunny weather. The rectal temperature will be greater than 40.5 °C and the patient will be in shock, but in the author's experience the commonest presenting sign is seizures; the excessive muscular activity will contribute to elevation of the core body temperature. Treatment involves the control of seizures, intravenous administration of methylprednisolone succinate and mannitol to reduce cerebral oedema and, if necessary, intubation and artificial ventilation. The gradual re-

duction of the body temperature may be achieved by wrapping the patient in cool wet towels. Fluid therapy will help treat shock and reduce the risk of subsequent renal failure (due to thermal renal damage and poor circulatory supply).

DYSAUTONOMIA

Neuronal degeneration of neurones in autonomic ganglia and other sites has been demonstrated in rabbits and hares with impactive mucoid enteropathy. Clinical signs tend to be non-specific and may include depression, anorexia, weight loss, accumulation of food material in the oral cavity and abdominal distension with palpable intestinal impaction. There may be a secondary inhalation pneumonia. At the time of writing, research funded by the BVA Welfare Foundation is investigating the condition. As in other species (horse, cat and dog) the aetiology remains uncertain. (Katherine Whitwell, personal communication).

GENERALIZED PARALYSIS AND COLLAPSE

Generalized weakness may be a late feature of many systemic diseases. Any infectious disease that can affect the CNS or musculoskeletal system can lead to similar signs. Generalized neuromuscular weakness may be attributable to myositis from infection with *Toxoplasma* or *Sarcocystis*. Paralysis has been seen as a feature of coccidiosis.

'Floppy rabbit syndrome'
This is a condition or group of conditions where affected rabbits suffer a paralysis of rapid onset affecting the limbs and notably the neck. Poisonous plants have been implicated in one instance and electrolyte disturbances have been suggested, but the aetiology is not yet known. In severe instances patients will die as a result of respiratory failure, but others may survive with supportive care.

There are anecdotal reports of myasthenia gravis in rabbits. The presentation is of a weak patient reluctant to move with no other apparent disease and a rapid response to intravenous edrophonium, a notable sign being erection of previously collapsed ears. Treatment with oral pyridostigmine and corticosteroids may be of benefit.

Metabolic disorders
Pregnancy toxaemia (see Chapter 6) in periparturient or pseudopregnant does may manifest as weakness and can progress to seizures and coma. The appropriate approach to ketosis is indicated. Hypocalcaemia may also occur in lactating does and can lead to weakness and recumbency, and intravenous adminis-

tration of a suitable calcium preparation to effect is indicated. Does with pyometra may present with hindlimb paralysis as emboli from septic foci in the abdomen can pass in a retrograde direction into the spinal venous system.

Diabetic ketoacidosis may present as weakness or collapse. The diagnosis may be made on routine blood tests and many patients improve with the appropriate fluid therapy. Most cases do not require long-term insulin administration as dietary correction, ensuring sufficient fibre is ingested, is usually sufficient to maintain satisfactory blood glucose levels.

Muscular dystrophy resulting from a vitamin E deficiency has been reported following degradation of this vitamin in stored pelleted diet. As is discussed elsewhere in this volume, feeding an appropriate diet will preclude this problem. The feeding of poorly stored feed can also lead to signs of vitamin A deficiency where a variety of neurological signs such as ataxia, torticollis, paralysis and convulsions may occur.

LEAD POISONING

Rabbits are inclined to gnaw at almost anything they happen across in the course of their travels. In the house and garden environment this may include discarded sources of lead. The signs of poisoning tend to be vague, with depression, loss of appetite and weight loss. Abdominal radiography may reveal radiodense material in the gastrointestinal tract. Haematological examination of fresh blood smears may show a reticulocytosis with basophilic stippling of red blood cells. Treatment involves subcutaneous administration of calcium EDTA as in other species.

OPTIC NEUROPATHY

Optic neuropathy associated with demyelination has been created as a laboratory model, but in general practice one is much more likely to see glaucomatous optic neuropathy. Glaucoma may be defined as an optic neuropathy where elevated intraocular pressure (IOP) is a risk factor, rather than a disease where the primary concern is raised IOP. Ophthalmoscopy will allow direct visualization of the optic disc where cupping is a typical feature, indicating loss of axonal tissues. By the time the patient has been presented with the characteristic signs of glaucoma the optic nerve is usually irreparably damaged (Figure 7.7). Inherited glaucoma has been described in the New Zealand white rabbit. The intraocular pressure begins to rise within the first 3 months of life and causes loss of vision, though discomfort is not a clinical feature (see Chapter 8).

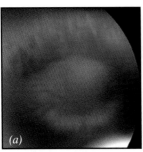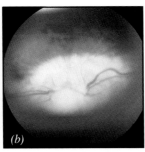

Figure 7.7: *(a) Glaucomatous optic neuropathy. (b) Normal optic disc for comparison.*

FURTHER READING

Hillyer EV (1994) Pet Rabbits. *Veterinary Clinics of North America (Small Animal Practice)* **24**, 24-25

Kunstyr I and Naumann S (1985) Head tilt in rabbits caused by pasteurellosis and encephalitozoonosis. *Laboratory Animal Science* **19**, 208-213

Manning PJ, Ringler DH and Newcomer CE (eds) (1994) *The Biology of the Laboratory Rabbit, 2nd edn.* Academic Press, New York

Tesluk G, Peiffer RL & Brown D (1982) A clinical and pathological study of inherited glaucoma in New Zealand white rabbits. *Laboratory Animals* **16**, 234-239

Weissenbock H, Hainfellner JA, Berger J, Kasper I and Budka H (1997) Naturally occurring Herpes simplex encephalitis in a domestic rabbit (*Oryctolagus cuniculus*). *Veterinary Pathology* **34**, 44-77

CHAPTER EIGHT

Ophthalmology

David Williams

INTRODUCTION

Relatively few conditions affect the rabbit eye and of those that do the majority of cases present as conditions involving the ocular adnexa. Conjunctivitis and dacryocystitis are perhaps the most common conditions presented, while uveitis, cataract and glaucoma are the main intraocular diseases encountered. Although few in number, these conditions affect a substantial number of rabbits and pose sufficient diagnostic and therapeutic challenges to be a significant problem in rabbit medicine.

While many accounts of ocular disease across the species begin with a discussion of the anatomy and physiology of the eye, the differences between the lagomorph and other, more familiar, mammalian eyes will here be introduced in the context of individual diseases. Similarly, techniques of ocular examination will not be covered in detail; classical techniques such as direct and indirect ophthalmoscopy and slit lamp biomicroscopy can readily be used when examining the rabbit eye without undue variation from those applied to other mammals.

CONJUNCTIVITIS

Mucoid or mucopurulent ocular discharge is a common finding in rabbits. The key feature in the investigation of such a case is defining whether the discharge merely signals a localized conjunctivitis, or whether it is the result of dacryocystitis, as discussed further below. The optimal technique used to differentiate between simple conjunctivitis and dacryocystitis is cannulation of the nasolacrimal duct. The rabbit nasolacrimal system is unusual in that there is only one ventrally placed nasolacrimal punctum. This is often quite deep in the inferior conjunctival sac and especially difficult to cannulate when there is concurrent severe conjunctivitis with hyperaemic and hyperplastic conjunctivitis (Figure 8.1). Digital presure ventrally on the lower eyelid causes the lips of the punctum to 'pout', facilitating introduction of a fine nasolacrimal cannula (Figure 8.2). Easy flushing without the appearance of purulent material around the cannula suggests that dacryocystitiis is not present.

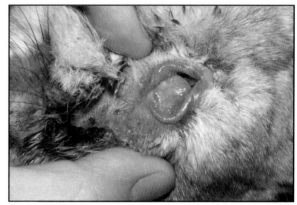

Figure 8.1: Conjunctivitis and nasolacrimal duct obstruction. Note the red conjunctiva with mild chemosis, rendering nasolacrimal cannulation difficult, and the fur loss from chronic epiphora. Note also that there is no purulent discharge, showing that while nasolacrimal duct function is compromised there is no dacryocystitis.

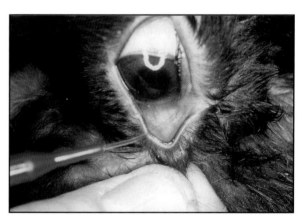

Figure 8.2: Cannulation of the single ventral punctum of the nasolacrimal duct. Here the lid is being pulled out to expose the punctum while in other cases it can be more beneficial to press upwards on the lower lid, everting the lips of the punctum.

Conjunctivitis may be caused simply by irritation from dust arising from poor quality hay or straw or may have an infectious aetiology. Distichia or ectopic cilia have not been reported causing ocular irritation and inflammation in the rabbit, although a single ectopic cilium has been noted from the nictitating membrane conjunctiva in more than one rabbit by the author and colleagues. As such abnormalities can occur, close examination is always necessary in a refractory case of ocular surface irritation or inflammation. The range of normal bacterial flora of the conjunctival sac is important to consider when taking a diagnostic approach to infective conjunctivitis and dacryocystitis (Okuda and Campbell, 1974).

Pasteurella spp. are often considered to be the most common bacterial pathogens in the rabbit, but *Staphylococcus aureus* should not be overlooked. Indeed, in a survey of staphylococcal disease in rabbits, over 60% had nasal exudate with conjunctivitis (Snyder *et al.*, 1976). A more recent study showed *Staphylococcus* sp. isolated from 40% of rabbits with ocular infection, while *Pasteurella* only occured in 12% (Cobb, 1999). Blepharoconjunctivitis with mucopurulent ocular discharge and eyelid thickening and crusting was reported associated with localized *Staphylococcus aureus* infection in one pregnant doe (Millichamp and Collins, 1986) in which immune compromise associated with the periparturient state was probably a significant factor precipitating the ocular infection. In that case, topical and parenteral gentamicin was curative. In another report an autogenous vaccine ameliorated ocular signs in rabbits with staphylococcal conjunctivitis (Hinton, 1977).

Haemophilus has also been reported as a pathogen causing conjunctivitis in the rabbit (Srivastava *et al.*, 1986). In that study the *Haemophilus* species isolated was also pathogenic to the normal rabbit eye unlike commensal flora incidentally isolated from many diseased eyes. The agent giving rise to ocular signs seen most comonly in wild rabbits is, however, not a bacterium but a virus, that of myxomatosis. The purulent white discharge seen with periocular swelling in myxomatosis (Figure 8.3) is probably not due to the virus itself but to date it is unclear exactly which organisms are involved. The immunosuppression caused by the viral infection probably accounts for the substantial conjunctival and palpebral lesions (probably caused by *Staphylococcus* or *Pasteurella*).

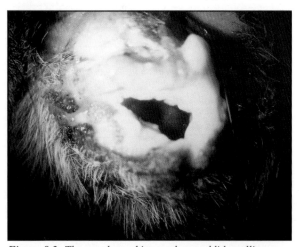

Figure 8.3: *The purulent white exudate and lid swelling characteristic of myxomatosis, here in a wild rabbit.*

As with conjunctivitis in other species, while bacteriological investigation is the first diagnostic step to take, cytology and the Schirmer tear test are also potentially useful diagnostic techniques in the evaluation of a rabbit eye with conjunctival reddening or mucoid discharges. Culture and sensitivity of a bacteriological sample take up to 3 days but cytology with Gram staining helps to define what class of bacteria are present, allowing the immediate choice of an appropriate antibiotic.

An example of the use of cytology is that of syphilitic ocular inflammation. Blepharitis in the rabbit may be associated with rabbit syphilis caused by the spirochaete *Treponema cuniculi*. The organism, and thus the condition, is transmitted to the neonates by the genitally infected dam (Harkness and Wagner, 1989). Diagnosis is made by demonstrating the spirochaete on a conjunctival scrape; this is best achieved with dark field illumination. Treatment is by injectable penicillin G at 40,000 IU/kg given three times, at 7-day intervals. Since ß-lactam antibiotics can cause fatal dysentery in rabbits, this treatment should be stopped should any diarrhoea occur, although this is unusual with parenterally rather than orally administered antibiotic (see Chapter 11). Squamous cell carcinoma can mimic the signs of treponemal blepharitis (Bagley and Lavach, 1985), although cytology readily shows the difference.

It might be considered strange that the Schirmer tear test was mentioned above, since keratoconjunctivitis sicca does not appear to occur often in rabbits. It is, however, only a lack of investigation that has resulted in so low a knowledge level with regard to normal and pathological lagomorph tear production. One study has reported Schirmer tear test values of on average 5.3 ± 2.9 mm/min in one study with a range from 0 mm/min to 15 mm/min in 142 apparently normal eyes (Abrams *et al.*, 1990). Breed differences accounted for the wide variation in this study but while it might be supposed that larger breeds would have the higher readings, the study showed Netherland dwarf rabbits to have an unusually high reading of 12.0 ± 2.5 mm/min. At the other end of the spectrum, the lowest value in normal rabbits was 0 mm/min. The Schirmer tear test, then, is probably a useful ancilliary test in a rabbit with ocular discharge or a red painful eye, but is not particularly useful at defining whether keratoconjunctivitis sicca is the pathological condition occurring in an eye. The Phenol Red Thread Test (Brown *et al.*, 1996) may be useful in rabbits but a normal range for this species has not, as yet, been published.

DACRYOCYSTITIS

This is a very important condition in the rabbit. The tortuous path of the nasolacrimal duct from the single nasolacrimal punctum through the lacrimal and maxillary bones to the distal recess of the external nares is one factor accounting for the propensity to develop duct obstruction and consequent epiphora (see Chapter 2). Another important factor is that the duct lies in close proximity to the root of the molar teeth, and more particularly the long roots of the incisors. Dental problems are, thus, a common cause for nasolacrimal duct obstruction and dacryocystitis (Crossley, 1996). Given the prevalence of dental disease in captive rabbits with nutritional hyperparathyroidism-related dental and facial bone abnormalities (Harcourt-Brown, 1996), it is understandable that nasolacrimal duct obstruction should be so common.

Sudden duct narrowing, with or without dental disease, results in specific sites where material can cause obstruction even without frank infection (Burling *et al.*, 1991; Marini *et al.*, 1996). Obstruction can be caused by sterile oil droplets in which case epiphora alone is noted (see Figure 8.1) (Marini *et al.*, 1996) or with infected purulent material giving dacryocystitis (Figure 8.4) (Petersen-Jones and Carrington, 1988). In infectious cases purulent material can be expressed from the nasolacrimal punctum with pressure just ventral to the punctum (Figure 8.5). Cannulation of the nasolacrimal canaliculus and flushing with sterile saline gives both the diagnosis, as purulent material is expelled, and the treatment, as the duct is cleared. Culture of nasolacrimal flushes from affected rabbits in one study (Marini *et al.*, 1996) showed a wide range of organisms including *Neisseria*, *Moraxella*, *Bordatella*, *Streptococcus viridans*, *Oligella urethralis* as well as *Pseudomonas*. These animals were affected by epiphora rather than dacryocystitis. Which of these organisms were part of the normal flora is not clear since the same organisms were found in nasolacrimal flushes from unaffected rabbits. *Pasteurella multocida*, the most frequently isolated organism in an earlier study of dacryocystitis, (Petersen-Jones and Carrington, 1988) was not detected. As was noted above, *Pasteurella* is not necessarily the most important organism in lagomorph external ocular infection, even if veterinary scientific folklore would suggest that to be the case!

ABERRANT CONJUNCTIVAL OVERGROWTH

An unusual abnormality unique to the rabbit is an aberrant overgrowth of conjunctiva giving an appearance similar to that of ankyloblepharon (Figure 8.6). The condition is poorly reported in the literature, and is described with a variety of different names and with a number of different suggestions as to its aetiology (Matros *et al.*, 1986; Bauck, 1989; Dupont *et al.*, 1995). While some suggest this is a congenital defect it can, however, first manifest itself in adult animals. A fold of conjunctival tissue arises from the limbus and appears at first examination as if a limbal keratitis was occurring. The tissue is, however, non-adherent to the cornea and may appear as a thin annulus or cover a considerable portion of the ocular surface. Surgical removal results in recurrence of the aberrant tissue, while suturing the fold back to the sclera, or using topical cyclosporin after surgery, prevents permanent visual impairment. Histology of resected tissue shows no inflammatory changes while special stains have demonstrated aberrant contractile elements in the leading edge of the conjunctiva (Miller and Murphy, personal communication). The aetiology of the condition is unknown.

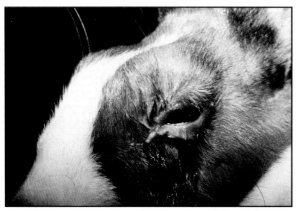

Figure 8.4: Dacryocystitis. The chronicity of the condition has led to palpebral inflammation. In many cases purulent discharge similar to that seen in Figures 8.3 and 8.5 is the only sign of dacryocystitis.

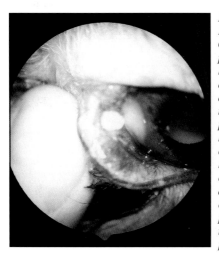

Figure 8.5: Dacryocystitis. Often upward pressure on the lower lid will expel purulent exudate from the nasolacrimal punctum. Note here also that conjunctival hyperaemia and corneal opacity are present, caused by pressure from the firm purulent focus.

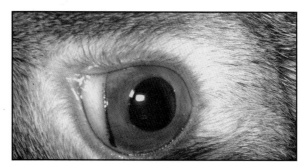

Figure 8.6: Aberrant conjunctival overgrowth. Here vision is not markedly compromised while in more severe cases the conjunctiva can grow to occlude almost the entire corneal surface.

DISEASES OF THE NICTITATING MEMBRANE

While prolapse of the gland of the nictitating membrane is common in the dog, only one report exists of a similar condition in the rabbit (Figure 8.7) (Roxburgh *et al.*, 1998. This documents a series of four rabbits in which frank prolapse or protrusion of the nictitans gland was seen in association with clinically and histologically determined hyperplasia. Other diseases of the nictitating membrane would include neoplasia, but this has yet to be reported in the veterinary literature.

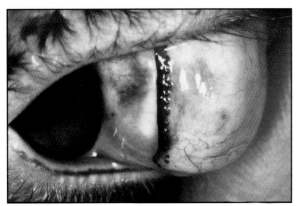

Figure 8.7: Prolapse of the deep gland of the nictitating membrane. Courtesy of Dr Gerlinde Janssens.

ORBITAL DISEASE

The most common orbital disease of rabbits is the retrobulbar abscess (Figure 8.8). Since these contain white or creamy-yellow pus they have generally been assumed to be caused by *Pasteurella multocida*. This may not necessarily be the case, as was shown above for dacryocystitis. The majority of them are related to dental disease. Infected molar tooth roots which are retropulsed into the orbit can readily lead to an orbital abscess, and a curative result in such a case is rarely achieved (see Chapter 13).

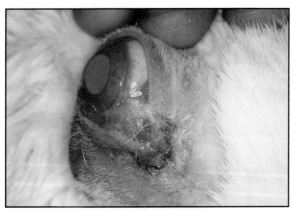

Figure 8.8: Retrobulbar abscessation leading to gross exophthalmos.

A large ventral retrobulbar venous sinus exists in the rabbit and because of this caution is necessary when performing an enucleation. Little problem occurs if pressure haemostasis is applied for a few minutes after removal of the globe, but unless haemorrhage is anticipated significant problems can occur during surgery.

CORNEAL LESIONS

Corneal epithelial dystrophy has been reported in the rabbit as peripheral areas of epithelial thinning and hyperplasia (Port and Dodd, 1983). Another report has described plaque-like paracentral granular stippling in American Dutch belted rabbits with irregularly thickened epithelial basement membrane demonstrated histologically (Moore *et al.*, 1987). Lipid keratopathy has, perhaps not suprisingly, been documented in rabbits fed cholesterol-rich diets to mimic human atherosclerotic disease (Fallon *et al.*, 1988) but also in rabbits fed a maintenance diet consisting of 10% fishmeal (Sebesteny *et al.*, 1985) and in one pet rabbit fed a predominantly milk-based diet (Gelatt, 1977).

UVEITIS

Uveitis in the rabbit may be caused by bacteria presumed to be seeded into the eye during a septicaemic episode. Characteristic signs are flare or frank hypopyon, synechiae and possibly also secondary cataract formation (Figure 8.9). Other cases are characterized by large iridal abscesses in eyes with panophthalmitis (Figure 8.10). While such cases of uveitis are seen on occasion, a more common presentation is that of a solitary white mass with, but more often without, other more overt signs of intraocular inflammation (Figure 8.11). These cases were previously thought also to be manifestations of *Pasteurella*, but recently have been shown to be a phacoclastic uveitis with a fascinating and unusual pathogenesis, as described below.

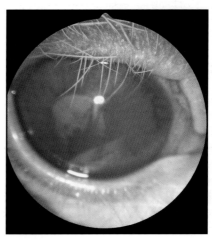

Figure 8.9: Anterior uveitis associated with intraocular Pasteurella multocida *reaching the eye by the haematogenous route. Note corneal oedema, hypopyon, flare and posterior synechiae.*

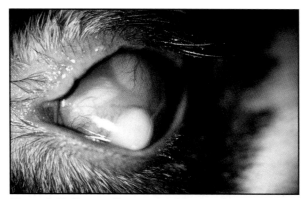

Figure 8.10: Pasteurella-*associated intraocular abscessation. Note that here the abscesses have exerted so much pressure on the cornea that perforation is imminent.*

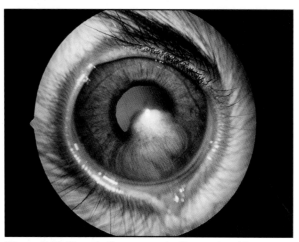

Figure 8.11: Encephalitozoon cuniculi-*associated lens-induced uveitis, showing the characteristic white iridal mass, here extending into the pupil and accompanied by iridal neovascularization. Courtesy of Dr SM Crispin.*

The microsporidian parasite, *Encephalitozoon cuniculi*, has for some time been known to cause cataract and lens capsule rupture in rabbits. It would appear that this protozoan enters the lens while it is developing *in utero*, and eventually leads to capsular rupture with or without cataract. Release of lens material into the anterior chamber leads to a phacoclastic uveitis. The only treatment for such an intraocular inflammation is lens removal, ideally by phacoemulsification, although albendazole has also been suggested to treat the parasitic infection itself.

GLAUCOMA

Glaucoma is inherited in the New Zealand White (NZW) rabbit and, given that the recessive *bu* gene occurs in pet rabbits of the NZW strain together with other white breeds, the same condition is seen in pet rabbits. The inherited glaucoma in the NZW rabbit has been well researched (Hanna *et al.*, 1962; Kolker *et al.*, 1963). Early in life, *bu/bu* homozygotes have normal intraocular pressure (15–23 mmHg), but at 1–3 months of age the pressure rises to between 26 and 48 mmHg

(McMaster, 1960). The eyes become buphthalmic with cloudy corneas (Figure 8.12) but, while vision is lost at this stage, the eyes do not appear painful. This may be because of nociceptive nerve fibre damage occurring as the globe expands. Over the next several months, intraocular pressure often returns to normal levels, since elevated pressure causes degeneration of the ciliary body which significantly reduces aqueous production. These affected eyes are characterized histologically by classical pectinate ligament dysplasia (Lee, 1968; Tesluk *et al.*, 1982). Medical treatment for this condition (Vareilles *et al.*, 1980) is rarely effective or necessary. The *bu* gene is a recessive trait which is also known to be semi-lethal in heterozygote animals, with the production of small litters of unthrifty kits.

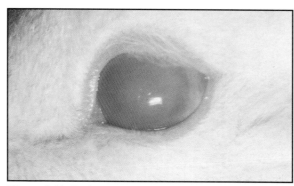

Figure 8.12: Early stages of glaucoma in a bu/bu *rabbit. Note the corneal oedema. There is little globe enlargement at this early stage, little episcleral congestion and no obviously detectable pain.*

POSTERIOR SEGMENT DISEASE

The retina of the rabbit is merangiotic, with a horizontal band of nerve fibres, normally myelinated and thus appearing white, with associated blood vessels (Figure 8.13). From a teleological perspective, it might be argued this leaves a horizontal band dorsal to the nerve fibres and blood vessels to be taken up by a horizontal photoreceptor-rich macula-like region. This, combined with the lateral eye placement in this species, allows the rabbit to have a relatively high level of resolution in a band around the entire horizon, in order to identify advancing predators readily from any direction.

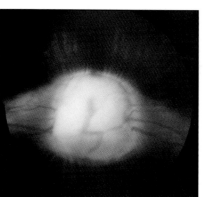

Figure 8.13: The normal merangiotic fundus of the rabbit.

The only spontaneous posterior segment disease commonly recognized in the rabbit is coloboma of the optic disc. These are not a significant problem but should be differentiated from the normally deep pit in the centre of the optic disc.

REFERENCES

Abrams KL, Brooks DE, Funk RS and Theran P (1990) Evaluation of Schirmer tear test in clinically normal rabbits. *American Journal of Veterinary Research* **51**, 1912-1913

Bagley LH and Lavach D (1985) Ophthalmic diseases in rabbits. *Californian Veterinarian* **49**, 7-9

Bauck L (1989) Ophthalmic conditions in pet rabbits and rodents. *Compendium on Continuing Education for the Practising Veterinarian* **11**, 258-268

Brown MH, Galland JC, Davidson HJ and Brightman AH (1996) The Phenol Red Thread Test in dogs. *Veterinary and Comparative Ophthalmology* **6**, 274-277

Burling K, Murphy CJ, Curiel JS, Koblick P and Bellhorn RW (1991) Anatomy of the rabbit nasolacrimal duct and its clinical implications. *Progress in Veterinary and Comparative Ophthalmology* **1**, 33-40

Cobb MA, Payne B, Allen WM and Pott JM (1999) A survey of the conjunctival flora in rabbits with clinical signs of superficial ocular infection. In: *Proceedings of the British Small Animal Veterinary Association Congress*, April, 1999, Birmingham, UK, p250. BSAVA, Cheltenham

Dupont C, Carrier M and Gauvin J (1995) Bilateral precorneal membranous occlusion in a dwarf rabbit. *Journal of Small Exotic Animal Medicine* **3**, 41-44

Fallon MT, Reinhard MK, DaRif CA and Schwoeb TR (1988) Diagnostic exercise: eye lesions in a rabbit. *Laboratory Animal Science* **38**, 612-613

Gelatt KN (1977) Corneal lipidosis in a rabbit fed milk. *Journal of the American Veterinary Medical Association* **171**, 887-889

Hanna BL, Sawin PB and Sheppars LB (1962) Buphthalmia in the rabbit. *Journal of Heredity* **62**, 294-299

Harcourt-Brown F (1996) Calcium deficiency, diet and dental disease in pet rabbits. *Veterinary Record* **139**, 567-571

Harkness JE and Wagner JE (1989) *The Biology and Medicine of Rabbits and Rodents. 3rd edn.* Lea and Febiger, Philadelphia

Hinton M (1977) Treatment of purulent staphylococcal conjunctivitis in rabbits with autogenous vaccine. *Laboratory Animals* **11**, 163-164

Kolker AE, Moses RA, Constant MA and Becker B (1963) The development of glaucoma in rabbits. *Investigative Ophthalmology* **12**, 316-321

Lee PF (1968) Gonioscopic study of hereditary buphthalmia in rabbits. *Archives of Ophthalmology* **79**, 775-778

McMaster PRB (1960) Decreased aqueous outflow in rabbits with hereditary buphthalmia. *Archives of Ophthalmology* **64**, 388-391

Marini RP, Foltz CJ, Kersten D, Batchelder M, Kaser W and Li X (1996) Microbiologic, radiographic and anatomic study of the nasolacrimal duct apparatus in the rabbit (*Oryctolagus cuniculus*). *Laboratory Animal Science* **46**, 656-662

Matros LE, Ansari MM and Van Pelt CS (1986) Eye anomaly in a dwarf rabbit. *Veterinary Medicine (Avian/Exotic Practice)* **3**, 13-14

Millichamp NJ and Collins BR (1986) Blepharoconjunctivitis associated with *Staphylococcus aureus* in a rabbit. *Journal of the American Veterinary Medical Association* **189**, 1153-1154

Moore CP, Dubielzig R and Glaza SM (1987) Anterior corneal dystrophy of American Dutch belted rabbits: biomicroscopic and histopathological findings. *Veterinary Pathology* **24**, 28-33

Okuda H and Campbell LH (1974) Conjunctival bacterial flora of the clinically normal New Zealand white rabbit. *Laboratory Animal Science* **24**, 831-833

Petersen-Jones SM and Carrington SD (1988) *Pasteurella* dacryocystitis in rabbits. *Veterinary Record* **122**, 514-515

Port CD and Dodd DC (1983) Two cases of corneal epithelial dystrophy in rabbits. *Laboratory Animal Science* **33**, 587-588

Roxburgh G, Boydell P and Genovese L (1998) Prolapse and hyperplasia of a third eyelid gland in 4 rabbits. *Journal of the British Association of Veterinary Ophthalmologists* **12**, 4

Sebesteny A, Sheraidah GAK and Trevam DJ (1985) Lipid keratopathy and atheromatosis in an SPF rabbit colony attributable to diet. *Laboratory Animals* **19**, 180-188

Snyder SB, Fox JG, Campell LH and Soave OA (1976) Disseminated staphylococcal disease in laboratory rabbits (*Oryctolagus cuniculus*). *Laboratory Animal Science* **26**, 86-88

Srivastava KK, Pick JR and Johnson PT (1986) Characterisation of a *Hemophilus* sp. isolated from a rabbit with conjunctivitis. *Laboratory Animal Science* **36**, 291-293

Tesluk G, Peiffer RL and Brown D (1982) A clinical and pathological study of inherited glaucoma in New Zealand white rabbits. *Laboratory Animals* **16**, 234-239

Vareilles P, Coquet P and Lotti VJ (1980) Intraocular pressure responses to antiglaucoma agents in spontaneous buphthalmic rabbits. *Ophthalmology Research* **12**, 2296-2302

CHAPTER NINE

Dermatoses

David H. Scarff

INTRODUCTION

Diseases of the skin and its appendages are common reasons for presentation of the rabbit to a veterinary surgeon. If this is to be a successful exercise, a similar approach is necessary to the one taken every day for canine and feline dermatoses, i.e. a diagnostic effort followed by specific treatment. As in much of small mammal medicine, however, the limitations imposed by financial considerations are of importance. Paradoxically, this increases the need for an accurate diagnostic effort from the outset.

This chapter considers the general approach to problems of the rabbit skin followed by a detailed account of different dermatoses, listed according to cause.

GENERAL APPROACH

To make the best use of information gained at history taking and initial examination, some knowledge of correct husbandry of the rabbit is essential. Many owners (not just children) are not very aware of the needs of the rabbit for appropriate housing and nutrition. Some owners believe they have a lot of knowledge but this may not all be accurate. The assessment of these factors is important in the accurate diagnosis and therefore successful treatment of rabbit dermatoses.

Rabbits may be kept in several different husbandry systems and for a number of different purposes. This may influence the incidence of some dermatoses; e.g. rabbits kept indoors ('house rabbits') are more likely to be exposed to cat fleas or to dermatophytes such as *Microsporum canis*. Rabbits kept in large groups are more likely to have contagious diseases but are less likely to be poorly fed. Pet rabbits kept outside in rural areas are more likely to be exposed to insect vectors of viral diseases such as myxomatosis.

A diagnostic approach consists of the following components:

- History taking
- General clinical examination
- Examination of the skin
- Differential diagnosis
- Special tests
- Firm diagnosis and treatment.

History
Careful history taking is essential for the accurate appraisal of any disease. This can be difficult when the animal is examined infrequently. Many small mammal consultations start with 'We found him like this.'

The first decision to be taken when gathering history about the pet rabbit is who to listen to. The 'owner,' usually a child, together with a parent or other adult, frequently accompanies the rabbit. Many adults do not accept that a child is capable of answering questions in this 'adult' environment and yet often are incapable themselves of supplying accurate information regarding husbandry. Furthermore, many adults would rather supply incorrect information than to admit this. If possible, the child should be involved, even if this does reveal the uncomfortable admission that they have been mentioning this problem for some time.

Initial questions should request information on basic husbandry of the rabbit:

- Breed, age and sex
- Length of time owned and source – pet shop, private breeder, etc.
- Type of housing – hutch indoors or outdoors, outbuilding, house, commercial housing (purpose-built or converted)
- Type of flooring e.g. wire or wooden
- Size of rabbit population and sex of other rabbits
- Other species in direct contact or sharing environment
- Method and frequency of cleaning hutch and type of cleaning agent
- Bedding and whether the rabbit eats it
- Foodstuffs provided, including supplements
- Type of water container – if in a commercial group, what hygiene measures are used for drinkers, etc.
- Is the environment protected against insect vectors of disease, such as mosquitoes? Do wild rabbits enter the garden? If so, do they look healthy?

Answers to these questions should allow some assessment of both the actual husbandry and level of knowledge of the owner.

The next step is to focus on the presenting complaint itself:

- What is the general health of the rabbit? Owners may be reluctant to dwell on this as they are keen to discuss the problem as they see it
- What is the problem that the owners are worried about?
- How long has it been noticed? (Not necessarily the same as 'how long has it been a problem?')
- Are any other rabbits affected? If so, are they in contact or just housed close by?
- Are any other species affected? This should include careful questions about the people who handle the rabbit without causing alarm about zoonotic disease at this stage
- What treatments (including proprietary drugs) have been used and with what success?
- Is the condition pruritic?
- Have any parasites been seen?
- If the pet is a house rabbit, are there cats or dogs in the same environment, and what flea control is practised?

General clinical examination

Unfortunately, many rabbits are presented in a stressed state (often in a cardboard box stuffed with straw or hay), which is not ideal, as observation of the animal at rest can give a useful idea of general health. In particular, signs of respiratory disease may be noted. Good restraint of the rabbit is essential for examination (see Chapter 1).

A full examination of the rabbit should be undertaken, even if the problem seems obvious. For example, clinical cheyletiellosis may be the consequence of underlying disease such as pasteurellosis. Underlying disease may interfere with a successful outcome, and stressful treatments such as dipping may lead to exacerbation of the underlying problem.

Examination of the oral cavity and dental arcade is of specific importance to some skin disorders, such as moist dermatitis and subcutaneous abscesses, and should be undertaken carefully. Likewise, careful examination of the respiratory system, including the nares and conjunctivae for signs of pasteurellosis, is important.

Examination of the skin

Complete examination of the skin should be undertaken, even if the dermatosis seems to be localized. Areas of particular importance include:

- The face, including the nares for nasal discharge and conjunctivae
- The ventral neck
- The pinnae and external ear canals
- The dorsum above the scapulae
- The feet, especially the footpads
- The external genitalia
- The perineum and tail fold.

Areas of scaling, changed colour (especially any blue-green pigmentation of fur), excoriation, alopecia or subcutaneous swellings should be noted. Examination of the coat with an illuminated hand lens may aid in the detection of external parasites (Figure 9.1).

Test	Technique	Indication
Skin scraping	Clip affected area carefully Moisten skin with liquid paraffin Scrape gently – avoid excessive trauma	Ectoparasites Dermatophytes
Acetate strip samples	Clip affected area carefully Apply strip several times Use fresh tape – more adhesive	Ectoparasites Dermatophytes Assessment of self-trauma
Fine-needle aspirate	Clip and clean lesion Use 21 G needle – exudate may be thick	Subcutaneous abscesses Possible neoplasia
Wood's lamp examination	Allow lamp to warm up Perform test in dark room Allow enough time to examine carefully	*Microsporum canis* only Not all strains fluoresce
Bacterial culture	Standard aerobic culture	Possible infection with *Pseudomonas* spp.
Fungal culture	Take plenty of hairs or use Mackenzie brush technique	Dermatophytes including *Trichophyton mentagrophytes* and *M. canis*
Skin biopsy	Sedation or general anaesthesia usually required	Possible neoplasia or infection with *Treponema* spp.

Figure 9.1: Special diagnostic tests for skin.

PARASITIC DERMATOSES

The skin parasites of the domestic rabbit are listed in Figure 9.2.

Group	Parasite
Insects	
Flies	Blowflies
Fleas	*Ctenocephalides felis, Spilopsylla cuniculi*
Lice	*Haemodipsus ventricosus*
Mites	
Fur mites	*Listrophorus gibbus* *Cheyletiella parasitovorax*
Sarcoptic mites	*Sarcoptes scabiei* var *cuniculi* *Notoedres cati*
Demodectic mites	*Demodex cuniculi*
Ear mites	*Psoroptes cuniculi*

Figure 9.2: Skin parasites of the domestic rabbit.

Flies

The presentation of a flyblown rabbit is a common occurrence in most veterinary practices in the summer months. Myiasis is always a distressing condition for patients, owners and clinicians. There is always some lack of care involved with myiasis, and it can develop rapidly.

Clinical signs

Rabbits are usually depressed, with skin disease initially focused on the perineum and tail fold (Figure 9.3). Alopecia is often present, and the skin may be eroded or even necrotic (Figure 9.4). Careful examination and exploration (for which anaesthesia may be required) often reveals blowfly larvae. It is important to examine for evidence of entry into body cavities as this worsens the prognosis.

Careful examination usually reveals evidence of underlying disease, including: dental disease, precluding adequate grooming; locomotor disease, including hindlimb paresis; and diseases of the digestive system resulting in diarrhoea and soiling of the perineum.

Diagnosis

Clinical signs and demonstration of fly larvae are usually adequate for diagnosis. The investigation and management of underlying disease is extremely important.

Treatment

Careful clipping and cleaning of affected skin and removal of all fly larvae is essential. Systemic antibiotics are sometimes necessary in severely affected rabbits. Following initial treatment, the use of insecticidal powders and sprays has been suggested; however, these should not be necessary if the underlying disease and husbandry problems are sorted out.

In the USA the larvae of flies of the genus *Cuterebra* may affect rabbits housed outdoors. These larvae develop in subcutaneous sites and are removed surgically.

Fleas

Rabbits may be affected by two types of flea. The commonest is *Ctenocephalides felis*, the cat flea. Less commonly, *Spilopsylla cuniculi*, the rabbit stick-tight flea, may be found, especially where wild rabbits are in contact with domestic rabbits. *S. cuniculi* is of particular significance as a possible vector of myxomatosis virus. In the USA rabbits may be infested with *Cediopsylla simples* (the common Eastern rabbit flea) and *Odontopsyllus multispinosus* (the giant Eastern rabbit flea).

Clinical signs

House rabbits sharing an environment with cats or dogs may pick up newly emerged *Ctenocephalides felis* fleas. These may be carried without clinical signs or they may cause pruritus. *S. cuniculi* fleas are usually found attached to pinnal margins, although they may

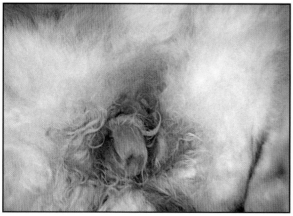

Figure 9.3: Perineum of rabbit with myiasis.

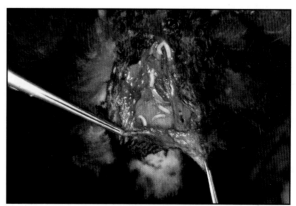

Figure 9.4: More severe case of myiasis. Note area of skin necrosis.

attach and feed on any part of the rabbit's skin. *Spilopsylla* spp. fleas may cause pruritus and tightly adherent crusts at the site of attachment.

Diagnosis
Flea faeces in the coat of a normal or pruritic rabbit are often the only clinical sign of infestation with *C. felis* fleas. This is not the case with rabbit fleas – demonstration of adult fleas is diagnostic of infestation with *S. cuniculi*.

Treatment
As with canine or feline flea problems, the eradication of *C. felis* infestation requires attention to the environmental stages and the adult fleas. If the house does not contain cats or dogs, then environmental control alone is often enough. If the household does contain cats or dogs with access to the outdoors, then the use of an adulticide together with environmental control may be necessary. There are no insecticidal products licensed for the rabbit. Pyrethrum-containing flea powders suitable for puppies or kittens have been recommended, although without environmental control their efficacy may be limited. Sprays containing fipronil should not be used as there have been incidents of adverse reactions in rabbits. Although these may represent overdosage or problems with inhalation of the vehicle, the use of 'spot-on' preparations is not recommended either. Imidacloprid has also been used in the rabbit, apparently without adverse effects, although it should be noted that this agent has no acaricidal properties.

The control of *S. cuniculi* fleas relies upon two measures: the control of attached adult fleas, and the prevention of future infestation. Adult fleas may be controlled either with pyrethrum-containing flea powders or by manual removal. Prevention of future infestation is best achieved by either screening of the rabbit hutch or by limiting access of wild rabbits to the garden.

Lice
Lice are uncommon causes of skin disease in the rabbit. Rabbit lice (*Haemodipsus ventricosus*) are of the sucking type, and heavy infestations may result in anaemia.

Clinical signs
Affected rabbits may be severely pruritic, although this is uncommon. Anaemic animals may be depressed and lethargic, and heavy infestations may result in scaling and crusting on the dorsal trunk.

Diagnosis
Lice or their eggs are usually demonstrated without difficulty. The eggs are larger than those of *Cheyletiella* spp. or *Listrophorus* spp. and are attached along most of the length of the egg.

Treatment
Pyrethrum-containing insecticidal powders are usually effective. Ivermectin injected at 200–400 µg/kg s.c. on three occasions at intervals of 2 weeks may also be effective.

Fur mites
Two types of fur mite are found in the pelage of the domestic rabbit – the true fur mite, *Listrophorus gibbus*, and the more surface-living *Cheyletiella parasitovorax*. The former are often spotted incidentally and may be carried with no clinical disease, sometimes in large numbers. Severe pruritus has, however, been reported associated with this parasite (Patel and Robinson, 1993). *Cheyletiella* spp. are more frequently associated with disease and have some zoonotic significance. Lesions in owners consist of pruritic erythematous papules on contact sites such as the arms and trunk. The parasites do not persist on humans once the affected rabbits are treated.

Clinical signs
Rabbits affected with either species of fur mite may present with no skin disease at all. Conversely, significant pruritus may be associated with small numbers of mites. Cheyletiellosis is often associated with severe scaling, especially on the dorsum (Figure 9.5). When pruritic disease is caused by *L. gibbus*, the most important signs are self-trauma and associated hair loss. Clinical cheyletiellosis is more likely in rabbits with concurrent illness.

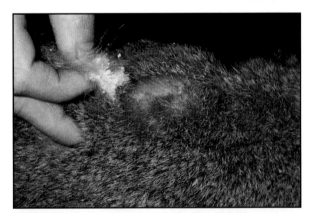

Figure 9.5: *Scaling of skin caused by* Cheyletiella parasitovorax.

Diagnosis
Demonstration of *L. gibbus* and *C. parasitovorax*, which may both occur in the same rabbit, is best achieved with the examination of acetate strip samples (Figure 9.6). In some cases superficial skin scrapings are required to demonstrate *Cheyletiella* spp., especially when present only in small numbers. Sometimes eggs only are found. The eggs of *Cheyletiella* spp. and *Listrophorus* spp. are similar and may be difficult to differentiate.

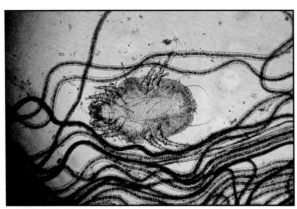

Figure 9.6: Adult female Cheyletiella parasitovorax *mite.*

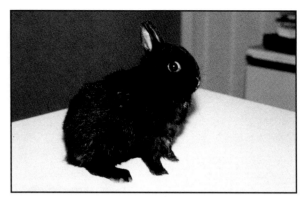

Figure 9.7: Dwarf rabbit carrying Demodex cuniculi *mites with minimal skin changes. Courtesy of R Harvey.*

Treatment

Both of these parasites seem to respond to ivermectin injections at the same dose rate suggested for lice infestation (200-400 µg/kg), and concurrent washing with 1 % selenium sulphide. If treatment does not solve the problem, asymptomatic carriers (which may include dogs or cats) or survival of parasites off the host must be suspected.

Sarcoptic mites

Rarely, rabbits are reported with infestation with sarcoptic mites, either *Sarcoptes scabiei* or *Notoedres cati*. The latter is rare in the UK and may not occur here even in cats, the normal host. Although all sarcoptic mites carry some zoonotic potential, they are more likely to cause a papular rash at contact sites on owners rather than true scabies, the pattern of disease caused by *S. scabiei var. hominis*.

Clinical signs

Pruritus and crusting around the head and pinnae are the most frequent clinical signs.

Diagnosis

Mites or their eggs must be demonstrated in deep skin scrapings from affected skin.

Treatment

Ivermectin injected at 200-400 µg/kg s.c. on three occasions at intervals of 2 weeks.

Demodectic mites

Demodectic mites have been reported rarely in the rabbit (Harvey, 1990) (Figures 9.7 and 9.8). Affected rabbits exhibited variable pruritus, although the pathological significance of the demodectic mites is unknown.

Ear mites

Psoroptes cuniculi, the rabbit ear mite, is the commonest ectoparasite of the rabbit. Infestations may occur some time after the last contact with another rabbit, and clinical disease may be initiated by concurrent stress.

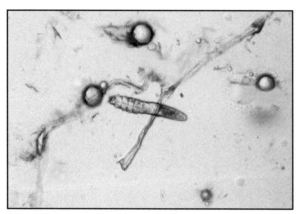

Figure 9.8: Adult Demodex cuniculi *mite from dwarf rabbit. Reproduced from Harvey (1990) with permission of the* Journal of Small Animal Practice.

Infected rabbits shed scale carrying large numbers of mites, which may survive for up to 3 weeks away from the host.

Clinical signs

Severe crusting and pain of the external ear canal and medial surface of the pinna are commonly found. Tightly adherent crusts are present in most cases, which leave bleeding erosions when removed. Curiously, only one pinna may be affected (Figure 9.9). Affected rabbits are often pruritic and rub at their ears. Secondary bacterial infection of crusted surfaces is common and may extend to cause otitis media.

Diagnosis

Demonstration of mites on examination of crusts taken from the pinna is usually straightforward (Figures 9.10 and 9.11). Large numbers of mites are often present. Removal of crusts may be painful, and so the minimum amount of material necessary should be taken.

Treatment

Ivermectin at 200-400 µg/kg injected subcutaneously on three occasions at intervals of 2 weeks is usually curative. Removal of crusts should not be attempted

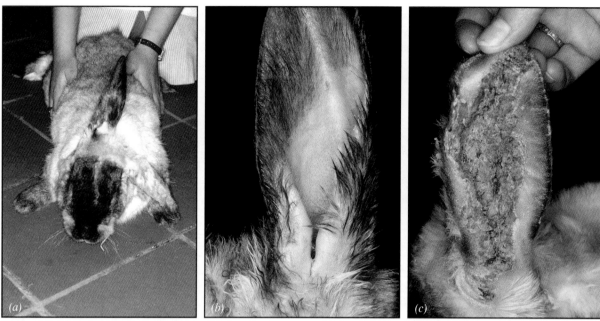

Figure 9.9: (a) Rabbit with Psoroptes cuniculi *infestation in one ear. (b) Normal ear. (c) Affected ear. Note tightly adherent crusts.*

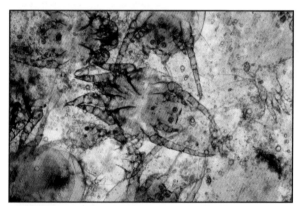

Figure 9.10: Adult male Psoroptes cuniculi *mite.*

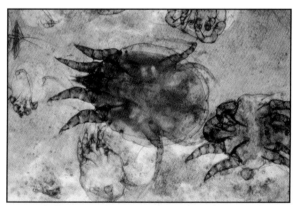

Figure 9.11: Adult female Psoroptes cuniculi *mite.*

as this is painful. The administration of ivermectin dissolved in mineral oil directly into the ear canal has been suggested, although this has little to offer over the injectable route. If the rabbit seems to be in pain from the otitis, then analgesics (e.g. carprofen, ketoprofen or meloxicam, see Chapter 12) should be administered for 2–3 days until the condition begins to resolve.

BACTERIAL DERMATOSES

Bacterial dermatoses may present in a variety of ways in the rabbit. The most common of these is the subcutaneous abscess. These lesions are associated with several different bacteria, including *Pasteurella multocida*, *Staphylococcus aureus* and various anaerobes.

Many of the bacterial dermatoses seen in rabbits are associated with bacteria endemic in the population, often carried with a minimum of obvious disease. The most frequent example of this is subclinical pasteurellosis. This may present in several ways, including respiratory disease ('snuffles'), conjunctivitis and subcutaneous abscesses. Subcutaneous abscesses are often associated with underlying disease, such as that affecting the dental arcade. For a more detailed discussion of dental disease see Chapter 13.

For the sake of clarity, the bacterial dermatoses are discussed by causative organism. It must be remembered, however, that mixed infections can occur.

Pasteurellosis
Most rabbits carry *Pasteurella multocida* in the nasal cavity asymptomatically. When stressed, clinical disease can occur (see Chapter 4). Subcutaneous abscesses are caused as an extension of a penetrating wound (including bite wounds), septicaemia or dental disease. Extension of disease to underlying bone may occur.

Clinical signs
Subcutaneous abscesses present as firm to fluctuant subcutaneous swellings. They may seem to be fixed to underlying structures, and although commonly found

around the head (Figure 9.12) and lower jaw, abscesses may occur in any site. Careful examination may reveal a penetrating wound. Other clinical presentations include mastitis in lactating does and skin disease at the medial canthus of the eye associated with chronic conjunctivitis and epiphora.

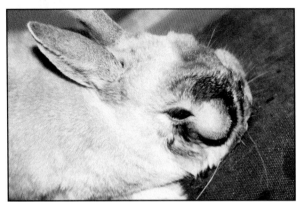

Figure 9.12: *Dwarf rabbit with a subcutaneous abscess secondary to pasteurellosis.*

Diagnosis
Fine-needle aspirates may be difficult to achieve unless a 21 G needle is used, as the exudate is very thick. Examination after staining with a rapid Romanowski stain reveals the causative organisms.

Examination for underlying disease is important, especially the assessment of the dental arcade. Unless underlying disease is identified and resolved, abscesses are likely to recur, whatever treatment is used. If a mixed infection is present, bacterial culture may be wise, including examination for anaerobic bacteria.

If underlying bone is thought to be involved, radiography is indicated to determine the extent of disease.

Treatment
The treatment of choice is the complete surgical excision of the abscess in its surrounding capsule. This may be extremely difficult, or impossible in the face of underlying dental disease. If this is not possible, then surgical opening of the abscess together with flushing and the use of topical or systemic antibiotic preparations may help. Such cases are, however, likely to recur, as are those with underlying bone or dental disease. See Chapter 11 for antibiotics suitable for use in the rabbit.

Staphylococcus aureus
Diseases caused by staphylococci may also present with several different clinical syndromes, from a highly fatal disease of neonatal rabbits to subcutaneous abscesses and an exudative dermatitis resembling impetigo. Mastitis and pododermatitis are also seen associated with this organism. Factors influencing the type of disease seen include the age when affected, concurrent disease or stress factors and the virulence of the strain of *S. aureus* seen. It would seem that phage group II strains may be the most virulent and may contain genes to produce epidermolytic toxins (Noble, 1989). A virulent rabbit biotype of *S. aureus* has been reported in Belgian rabbitries (Okerman *et al.*, 1984).

Clinical signs
Neonatal rabbits suffer from two specific patterns of staphylococcal disease – septicaemia and sudden death, and exudative dermatitis. Both of these may be associated with poor husbandry, and are most often reported from commercial rabbit-rearing units.

Diagnosis
Examination of swabs taken from rabbits affected with exudative dermatitis reveals the causative organism. Culture samples are necessary in septicaemic animals, and culture may allow the typing of the staphylococcal strains involved. Samples may be taken either as blood culture from adults or more easily from dead neonates.

Treatment
Systemic antibiotics are needed to control and prevent exudative dermatitis. This may not be an economic option in commercial units, where the culling of affected rabbits followed by disinfection of the premises and restocking may be necessary. If this is not done, the problem is likely to recur, as the causative organism is endemic in affected groups. Obviously, underlying problems such as overcrowding and poor hygiene in the premises should be improved to prevent recurrence.

Pseudomonas aeruginosa
This organism is responsible for a moist dermatitis, usually found on the ventral surface of the neck. This condition is predisposed by constant wetting of the affected skin, either by faulty drinking apparatus or due to dribbling secondary to dental disease ('slobbers'). The disease is noticeable by staining of the fur with blue-green pyocyanin pigment.

Clinical signs
There is moist dermatitis on the ventral neck area (dewlap) or flanks, which is often stained blue-green. The fur is often matted or clumped. The skin in affected areas is almost always wet.

Diagnosis
The clinical signs are nearly diagnostic in their own right. Bacterial culture may be helpful owing to the multiresistant nature of *Pseudomonas* spp. to many antibiotics.

Treatment
Clipping and cleaning of affected skin is important. Topical or systemic antibiotics may be used, although the condition is likely to recur if the underlying cause of wetting is not addressed.

Fusobacterium necrophorum

This anaerobic organism is the cause of an uncommon dermatosis affecting the rabbit.

Clinical signs

Fusobacterium necrophorum causes inflammation, erosion, ulceration or necrosis of skin, particularly around the head and neck. Subcutaneous abscesses may be seen.

Diagnosis

Direct smears may reveal the organism, although anaerobic culture is necessary to confirm the cause. Mixed infections may occur, and so aerobic culture should always be undertaken at the same time.

Treatment

Clipping, cleaning and surgical debridement, together with topical or systemic antibiotics are needed for successful treatment.

Treponema cuniculi

Venereal spirochaetosis, caused by *Treponema cuniculi* (see Chapter 6), is an uncommon dermatosis of the rabbit. Transmission is by direct contact, and owing to the rabbit's grooming practices, autotransmission to skin other than that of the genitalia is common.

Clinical signs

Vesicles, papules, oedema, erosion and crusting may be seen not only on the genitalia but also on the lips, face, eyelids, ears and paws. Lesions may be mistaken for early signs of myxomatosis, and if limited to scaling on the face may be confused with dermatophytosis.

Diagnosis

This may be difficult as *T. cuniculi* is difficult to culture, but examination of biopsy samples stained with silver stains or the demonstration of the organism in dark-ground microscopy examination confirms the diagnosis. Serological tests are available in some countries.

Treatment

The treatment of choice is penicillin injected at weekly intervals for 3 weeks. All affected and in-contact animals need to be treated, and the prognosis is good. Treatment with tetracycline or chloramphenicol is also effective.

Pododermatitis (sore hocks)

This condition is one of the most frustrating for the practitioner to deal with. Whereas bacteria are almost uniformly involved in this condition, other factors are needed to initiate disease. Predisposing factors include heavy body size, thin fur on the metatarsal pad, and wire flooring. Damp or soiled bedding may also contribute.

Clinical signs

Swollen metatarsal or metacarpal areas follow scaling and erosion of the volar surfaces. The swellings may be very large with necrotic centres (Figure 9.13).

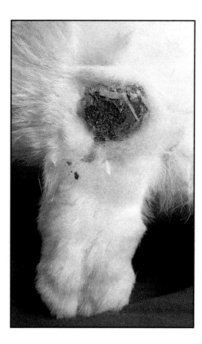

Figure 9.13: Rabbit with pododermatitis (sore hocks).

Diagnosis

The clinical signs are highly suggestive. *Staphylococcus aureus* may be isolated from culture samples in most cases.

Treatment

There are two facets to treatment of this condition. First, treatment will not be successful if the underlying factors are not identified and improved. Heavy rabbits (>5 kg) should not be housed on wire, and bedding should be changed regularly. Secondly, management of the lesions involves the application of topical anti-bacterial ointments such as mupirocin 2%. This is not licensed for use in this species. Severe lesions should be cleaned, debrided and, if possible, bandaged. Recurrence is common once disease is initiated, and the prognosis in severe cases is guarded. Surgical excision of the lesion should not be attempted. The skin overlying the metatarsus is firmly anchored to the underlying tissues and difficult to mobilise. Closure of the defect is therefore almost impossible.

VIRAL DERMATOSES

Myxomatosis

The most important viral dermatosis of the rabbit is myxomatosis (Figure 9.14) caused by a poxvirus. Myxomatosis is endemic in rabbit populations in South America. It was introduced into Australia in the 1950s to help control the rabbit population, and rapidly increased. The virus was then accidentally

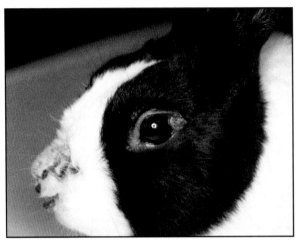

Figure 9.14: Vaccinated rabbit with chronic form of myxomatosis.

introduced into Europe, where it nearly eradicated the wild rabbit population. The disease is still endemic in wild populations of rabbits in Europe, although its virulence varies.

Insect vectors spread the myxoma virus. These include mosquitoes and the rabbit stick-tight flea, *Spilopsylla cuniculi*. Depending upon the virulence of the virus, several clinical syndromes occur, including a peracute infection that is invariably fatal, widespread skin tumour production and a temporary papillomatous condition in partially immune rabbits. A respiratory form of the disease occurs in France, spread by direct contact. An unusual variant of this disease occurred in recently depilated Angora rabbits, where multiple cutaneous papules and plaques appeared in the area that had been depilated. These lesions progressed to become necrotic and haemorrhagic. The disease was not highly fatal, and most rabbits recovered spontaneously (Ganière *et al.*, 1991). Various vaccines are available around the world. In the UK the only one available is a heterologous vaccine derived from Shope fibroma virus. This is variably successful, the efficacy being increased if the vaccine is partially injected intradermally.

Clinical signs
In acute cases rabbits are lethargic, febrile and depressed. Oedema of the ears, lips, eyes, genitalia and anus is present, and the disease rapidly progresses to death. In less virulent strains, skin tumours are produced in large numbers. These may regress spontaneously, although affected rabbits may be predisposed to respiratory infection or pasteurellosis.

Diagnosis
In the acute form of the disease, the clinical signs are diagnostic. In the early stages the disease may resemble venereal spirochaetosis, but the true diagnosis is soon apparent. In subacute or chronic forms, a biopsy is diagnostic in samples with intact epidermis.

Treatment
Treatment for myxomatosis is generally unsuccessful but some rabbits may recover after intensive nursing care. If an attempt at treatment is to be made, it is important to discuss this fully with the owner so that they appreciate the difficulties involved, and the prolonged duration of treatment that may be required. Rabbits should be maintained at a high environmental temperature (21–22 °C) during treatment. Fluid therapy and nutritional support are required, together with good nursing care – e.g. cleaning of the eyes and nares. Antibiotics are needed to prevent secondary infections. After recovery, skin tumours may still be present, and if necessary these can be excised. Since acute myxomatosis may cause considerable distress to the rabbit, and the likelihood of successful treatment is poor, clinicians should give careful consideration to all factors before embarking on a course of treatment.

Rabbits with subacute disease may recover spontaneously, but antibacterial treatment to prevent secondary respiratory infection is wise. Vaccination and screening for insect vectors are helpful in reducing the incidence of the disease.

Rabbit pox
This unusual infection of domestic rabbits is caused by a poxvirus related to the vaccinia virus. Initially rabbits are febrile and have a nasal discharge. This is followed by a generalized papular to nodular eruption. Extensive oedema of the face and perineum may be seen.

Shope papilloma virus
In the USA this oncogenic papovavirus is seen uncommonly. Like the Shope fibroma virus the Shope papilloma virus occurs naturally in the wild Brush rabbit and Cottontail rabbit (*Sylvilagus* spp.). It is spread by an insect vector and is responsible for the production of multiple cutaneous horns, especially on the face and eyelids. Spontaneous regression usually occurs within 12 months, but experimentally lesions may progress to squamous cell carcinoma.

Shope fibroma virus
This poxvirus is an uncommon cause of neoplasia in rabbits in the USA. Lesions consist of single or multiple firm subcutaneous nodules. Spontaneous regression may occur. This virus is the basis of the heterologous vaccines for myxomatosis.

FUNGAL DERMATOSES

Rabbits may suffer from dermatophytosis. There are two dermatophytes of significance in the rabbit, *Trichophyton mentagrophytes* and *Microsporum canis*. *T. mentagrophytes* is carried asymptomatically in the coat of many rabbits and *Microsporum canis* may infect rabbits in contact with cats and dogs. Whereas the latter is usually considered to be of more zoonotic significance, its pathogenicity in the fur of a paratenic host is unknown. *T. mentagrophytes* is more likely to cause zoonotic disease when carried by a rabbit than by a dog or cat.

Owners are often worried about the zoonotic significance of dermatophytosis in small mammals. These fungi are undoubtedly of some risk, although most people who become infected are predisposed in some way (e.g. atopic, immunosuppressed). In most cases the risk seems to be slight, although it is wise to limit an owner's contact with known infected animals, especially if the owner is a child.

Clinical signs
Trichophyton mentagrophytes may be carried asymptomatically in the coat of the rabbit. This may follow clinical disease, although in many cases this is inapparent. Clinical disease for both dermatophytes found in the rabbit is essentially similar. Scaling, crusting and alopecia with some pruritus are found. Usually the bridge of the nose is affected, together with the eyelids, ears and paws. Occasionally widespread disease is found. Broken hairs may be found on close examination, and these should be collected for fungal culture.

Diagnosis
Fungal culture is the test of choice for diagnosis. Examination by Wood's lamp may be useful in infections with *Microsporum canis*, although not all strains fluoresce. *Trichophyton* sp. does not fluoresce at all.

Treatment
Griseofulvin treatment at 25–50 mg/kg sid is the treatment of choice. It must, however, be remembered that this drug is unlicensed in the rabbit. It is also highly teratogenic and so must not be used in breeding does. Owners should handle griseofulvin carefully. Treatment should be continued until clinical signs have resolved. All in-contact rabbits should be treated. Topical enilconazole has also been used with success. Itraconazole has also be used at 10 mg/kg sid for 15 days, but it is expensive and unlicensed for use in the rabbit.

Clipping of the haircoat may be useful; although clipped hair should be disposed of by burning. From experiences in the cat, close clipping may increase the severity of clinical disease.

DERMATOSES CAUSED BY BEHAVIOUR

In the breeding season does may pluck hair from the dewlap area to line their nests. This may also occur in non-pregnant does, and such rabbits may be presented for alopecia. If excessive amounts of hair are removed and swallowed, hairballs may occur.

Barbering of hair by dominant rabbits may happen when rabbits are housed in groups. Environmental enrichment can help resolve this problem. If the rabbits are housed in a large enclosure, adding objects such as tubes and boxes may be helpful. If this fails and the barbering is severe, then separation of the rabbits may be necessary.

DERMATOSES CAUSED BY NUTRITION

Nutritional dermatoses are uncommon in the rabbit, although alopecia, scaling and coat depigmentation have been produced experimentally in animals on diets deficient in zinc or copper.

MISCELLANEOUS DERMATOSES

Congenital dermatoses
Congenital dermatoses including hereditary alopecia and cutaneous asthenia (Harvey *et al.*, 1990) have been reported in the rabbit. In cutaneous asthenia the skin has increased extensibility and is easily torn (Figures 9.15 and 9.16). Electron microscopy shows disorganization and variability in size of the collagen bundles (Figure 9.17).

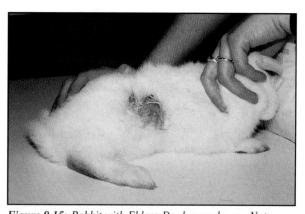

Figure 9.15: *Rabbit with Ehlers-Danlos syndrome. Note easily torn skin. Courtesy of R Harvey.*

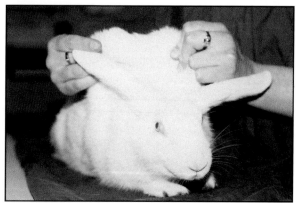

Figure 9.16: *Rabbit with Ehlers-Danlos syndrome showing excessive skin extensibility. Courtesy of R Harvey.*

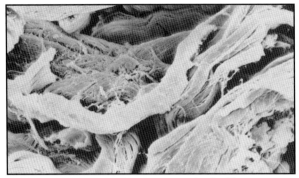

Figure 9.17: Electron photomicrograph of rabbit in Figure 9.15 showing disorganized collagen bundles. Reproduced from Harvey et al. (1990) with permission of The Veterinary Record.

Seborrhoeic dermatosis

Seborrhoea of the skin surrounding the scent glands lateral to the anogenital line is occasionally a problem. Mild antiseborrhoeic shampoos are usually helpful.

Seasonal dermatoses

Rabbits are occasionally presented with disorders of seasonal moulting. Such rabbits may have patches of retained telogen coat and patches of fur at different lengths. This is a problem that occurs more frequently in elderly rabbits. Careful grooming and attention to husbandry is usually helpful.

Urine scalding

Urine scalding of the perineal region may occur in rabbits housed in unsanitary conditions. Affected skin is moist and excoriated. This problem may be exacerbated if rabbits are obese or have locomotor disease (see Chapter 6).

Frostbite

If rabbits are suddenly exposed to very cold weather they may experience frostbite. Typically, this presents as necrosis of the pinnal margins and tip.

Neoplastic disease

Spontaneous cutaneous neoplasms are rare in the domestic rabbit. Those most frequently found are the lipoma and papilloma. In the USA the oncogenic viruses Shope papilloma virus and Shope fibroma virus are found uncommonly in domestic rabbits, but are endemic in wild rabbit populations.

Other neoplasms seen in the rabbit include squamous cell carcinoma, trichoepithelioma and basal cell tumour.

Subcutaneous lymphoma has also been reported, and may be diagnosed by the examination of fine-needle aspirates.

REFERENCES AND FURTHER READING

Brown SA and Rosenthal KL (1997) *Self-Assessment Colour Review of Small Mammals.* Manson, London

Collins BR (1987) Dermatologic disorders of common small nondomestic animals. In: *Dermatology,* ed. GH Nesbitt, pp. 235-295. Churchill Livingstone, New York

Ganière JP, Gourreau J-M, Montabord D *et al.* (1991) Myxomatosis of the depilated Angora rabbit. A preliminary study. *Veterinary Dermatology* **2,** 11-16

Harvey RG (1990) *Demodex cuniculi* in dwarf rabbits (*Oryctolagus cuniculus*). *Journal of Small Animal Practice* **31,** 204-207

Harvey RG, Brown PF, Young RD and Whitbread TJ. (1990) A connective tissue defect in two rabbits similar to the Ehlers-Danlos syndrome. *Veterinary Record* **126,** 130-132

Hillyer EV (1997) Dermatologic diseases. In: *Ferrets, Rabbits and Rodents: Clinical Medicine and Surgery,* ed. EV Hillyer and KE Queensbury, pp. 212-219. WB Saunders, Philadelphia

Noble WC (1989) Bacterial skin infections in domestic animals and man. In: *Advances in Veterinary Dermatology, Vol. 1,* eds. C von Tscharner and REW Halliwell, pp. 311-326. Baillière Tindall, London

Okerman L (1988) *Diseases of Domestic Rabbits,* pp. 40-52. Blackwell, Oxford

Okerman L, Devriese LA, Maertens L, *et al.* (1984) Cutaneous staphylococcosis in rabbits. *Veterinary Record* **114,** 313-315

Patel A and Robinson KJE (1993) Dermatosis associated with *Listrophorus gibbus* in the rabbit. *Journal of Small Animal Practice* **34,** 409

Paul-Murphy J and Moriello K (1995) Skin diseases of small mammals. In: *Handbook of Small Animal Dermatology,* ed. K Moriello and I Mason, pp. 245-253. Elsevier, Oxford

Scott DW, Miller WH Jr, and Griffin CE (1995) Dermatoses of pet rodents, rabbits and ferrets. In: *Muller and Kirk's Small Animal Dermatology,* pp. 1153-1161. WB Saunders, Philadelphia

CHAPTER TEN

Behaviour Problems

Sally O. Walshaw

INTRODUCTION

Before 1985 pet rabbits in the UK and USA usually lived in outdoor hutches. Interaction between rabbit and owner occurred mainly at feeding time. In a busy urban society, rabbits purchased in pet shops increasingly went to homes where outdoor hutches were neither available nor desired by the rabbits' owners. Unfortunately, owners were not always prepared to cope with undesirable rabbit behaviour in the house. As a result, some owners were abandoning their pet rabbits at animal shelters or, worse still, leaving them to fend for themselves in nature. Since 1988, the US House Rabbit Society has attempted to deal with this problem by establishing a network of rabbit foster care homes. In the UK the British Houserabbit Association, founded in 1996, is taking a leading role in educating veterinary surgeons and rabbit owners about these animals.

The problem of abandoned rabbits can best be addressed by providing their owners with detailed information about the normal behaviour of the domestic rabbit and methods of shaping their pets' behaviour. Strictly speaking, rabbits do not have behavioural problems; people have problems with house rabbits unless they devise ways of coping with the natural tendencies of the animal. The goal is to enable the house rabbit to achieve its potential as a delightful companion animal: clean, playful, and affectionate.

NORMAL RABBIT BEHAVIOUR

The domestic rabbit in the USA and Europe is descended from the European wild rabbit, *Oryctolagus cuniculus*. Detailed field observations of the wild European rabbit document behaviour that is very similar to that of domestic house rabbits. Many new rabbit owners expect the rabbit to be a placid animal, much like a stuffed toy. Actually, the rabbit is a very curious animal that actively explores its environment (Figure 10.1). As with dogs and cats, a house rabbit's life involves some mischief, especially during the first year. Puppies will chew on clothing, furniture and carpets; kittens will climb curtains and use their claws on furniture; rabbits will chew on household objects and dig in soft materials if given the opportunity.

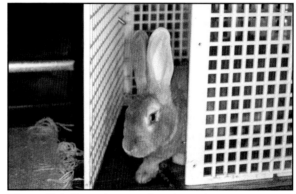

Figure 10.1: Preparing to explore the environment.

Activity

The mature rabbit, whether wild or domesticated, is normally active early in the morning and again in the late afternoon or early evening. Feeding, followed by resting, occurs primarily during, and particularly near the ends of, these two active periods. In the morning, the rabbit can play outside its pen, under supervision, while the family has breakfast. While the owners are busy at daytime tasks and children are at school, the rabbit has its natural nap. In nature, the wild rabbit often spends its long rest period in the warren. Consequently, the house rabbit adjusts readily to living part of the time in a pen or cage. The rabbit is playful in the early evening and family members can enjoy the rabbit's antics when the rabbit is allowed out of its pen.

During periods of activity, the rabbit hops about its territory, marking it with colourless (and odourless, to humans) droplets from small glands underneath its chin (Figure 10.2). A sexually intact rabbit may also mark its territory by spraying urine on objects or by leaving droppings here and there in an area. A rabbit will readily jump on to furniture, often climbing to a higher perch, and conversely explore various hiding places behind curtains and under chairs. A lively rabbit in a room or hallway may suddenly shake its head and then hop quickly across an open area while twisting its rear quarters in the air. The rabbit may also jump up and turn 180 degrees in the air before landing. A rabbit will play chase games with another rabbit or with its human owner, provided that the rabbit chases the human and not vice versa.

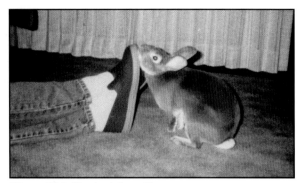

Figure 10.2: Territorial marking.

While moving about the house, the rabbit will investigate objects using its nose and mouth; it loves to chew. Picking up small objects and throwing them is a common behaviour of rabbits; it will move things with its nose, teeth, and front feet. A house rabbit may drag, for example, a toilet brush out of the bathroom and through the house! Furthermore, a rabbit, especially a sexually intact female, may dig extensive burrows if placed in an outside pen.

Social interaction

A social hierarchy is an important part of a rabbit's life. Rabbits kept together may become bonded, with mutual grooming and sleeping in contact with each other. A rabbit may enjoy 'grooming' the owner's hair (Figure 10.3). A house rabbit in a one-rabbit home may establish dominance over other members of the household, e.g. dogs, cats, and perhaps people. It signals its dominance quite differently from another companion animal, the dog. A dominant rabbit presents its face to a subordinate (rabbit or human) for grooming. Licking or nudging a person's hand or foot is one way a rabbit solicits petting from the owner. To a rabbit, being petted or groomed on its head signifies its dominance.

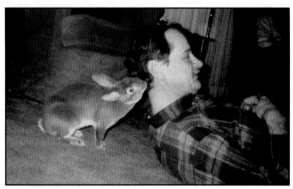

Figure 10.3: Hair grooming.

The behaviour of a house rabbit toward mild-mannered dogs and cats differs from the response of a wild rabbit to these predator species. If the dog or cat does not chase the rabbit, the rabbit will approach the dog or cat. The rabbit may then sniff the dog or

cat, nibble on its fur, or even mark the animal with its chin glands. Many pet dogs and cats will accept the presence of a house rabbit and learn to suppress their natural chase instincts (Figure 10.4). However, the rabbit should never be left unsupervised with carnivorous pets, such as dogs and cats. Some rabbits have an innate fear of ferrets, triggered even by their scent, that may complicate having these animals in the same household.

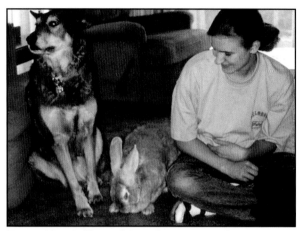

Figure 10.4: Rabbit and dog in harmony together.

Vocalization

One aspect of the rabbit's behaviour that makes it an attractive animal in urban housing situations is that it will not annoy the neighbours by barking. Although generally silent, rabbits are capable of making a variety of sounds. A soft humming noise from a male rabbit circling around the owner may be the prelude to a mating attempt with the owner's foot. A contented rabbit may quietly chatter its teeth while relaxing during a petting session. A rabbit that does not want to be disturbed may growl or hiss and rush toward an intruder with its neck extended, its tail held straight out, and its teeth bared. A very frightened or injured rabbit can emit a pitiful high-pitched scream. Stamping with the hind feet is the rabbit's way of signalling a perceived danger. Reluctance to move, sometimes accompanied by loud grinding of teeth, may signal pain.

Grooming

Grooming behaviour is a sign of good health in the rabbit, as it is for birds and other mammals. The rabbit licks its forepaws to clean its ears and face thoroughly and uses its tongue to preen its entire hair coat. Moulting occurs approximately four times a year in the house rabbit. Owners can help to prevent 'hairball' (trichobezoar) formation (and possibly fatal gastrointestinal obstruction) by frequent use of brushes or fine-tooth combs. Twice-daily small doses of an oral pet laxative may be indicated for therapeutic and/or preventive care of a rabbit diagnosed with trichobezoars.

GENERAL TRAINING TIPS

Treats

Rabbits relish various treat foods, e.g. sweetened dry breakfast cereal, fresh vegetables, and raisins (Figure 10.5). A plastic container of commercial sweetened breakfast cereal makes a rattling sound when shaken. This is quite useful in teaching a rabbit to come when its name is called. It is important to give the rabbit a tasty treat and appropriate regular foods every time it is returned to its primary housing area (large cage or rabbit-proofed room). A treat for the rabbit is also in order, during the training phase, after it has been lifted and carried.

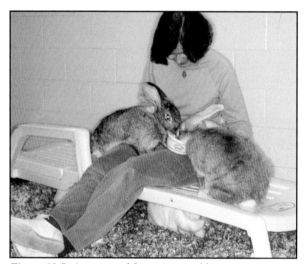

Figure 10.5: A treat used for training rabbits.

Physical interaction

Rabbits do not always enjoy being held on a person's lap. However, rabbits are affectionate and active, and winning their trust is not difficult. It is best, with a new rabbit, to interact with it on its level in a small room. The rabbit, by nature, is a prey animal, so techniques used in taming a wild or fearful horse work well with the rabbit. The new owner should sit quietly on the floor and read a book while the rabbit explores the room. The rabbit is a curious animal and will soon want to investigate the person who is sitting on the floor reading. Patience is essential when establishing trust with a rabbit. An owner should never let a rabbit know he or she is in a hurry. If the owner is relaxed, the process of becoming acquainted will be easier and quicker.

When the rabbit approaches the owner, the person may reach out slowly to pet it. Rabbits have relatively poor depth perception so it is not useful to offer one's hand for the rabbit to inspect as one would when meeting a dog. Mutual grooming in rabbits often involves the face. Therefore, the owner should stroke the rabbit slowly and gently on the head in front of the ears and around the eyes and cheeks, avoiding the ticklish muzzle.

Introducing a new rabbit

Newly introduced rabbits should have separate cages and meet each other for short play sessions, ideally in neutral territory, under careful supervision by the owner. A little chasing and hair-pulling are normal behaviours in this situation. However, the owner should be prepared to stop fights by stamping his/her feet, spraying the rabbit(s) with water, and using towels or heavy gloves to separate them, if necessary. Several months may elapse before the rabbits can be safely together. The stress of a car ride (including a trip through a car wash) has led to bonding between rabbits placed side by side in the back seat of the car. Male–female pairs, in which both rabbits have been neutered, have the highest success rate, but much depends on the rabbits' personalities.

Drinking

Training a rabbit to drink from a syringe is useful in case the rabbit ever needs oral liquid medication, such as certain analgesics and antibiotics. The training method takes advantage of the rabbit's attraction to sweet flavours. The owner mixes water with a generous amount of sugar and draws this solution into the syringe. The tip of the syringe is dipped first into water and then into granulated sugar. The sweetened tip of the syringe is offered to the rabbit to chew and the solution is administered slowly. Rabbits learn quickly and will readily drink children's flavoured oral medications from a syringe.

LITTER BOX TRAINING

Litter box training of a rabbit is generally accomplished fairly easily, even if the rabbit is an adult. A rabbit (especially if neutered) chooses a single area, in a corner or along a wall, for urination and most of its defecation. A litter box should be placed in the desired location in the rabbit's home cage or room (Figure 10.6). Food and water bowls are then positioned in the other corners. The litter box should be large enough for the rabbit to sit in comfortably and have sides over which the rabbit can jump easily.

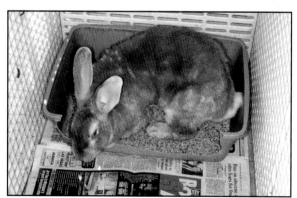

Figure 10.6: Rabbit using a litter box.

During the training phase, it is helpful to confine the rabbit, especially if it is young, most of the time to its main housing area. The young animal will enjoy brief (30 minutes) play and exploration sessions several hours apart in one small room of the house, e.g., a bathroom. Any newly acquired rabbit should be gradually (over a period of weeks) allowed to explore safe areas of the home. The day's designated foods should be divided into as many portions as there are play sessions. During the training phase, feed the rabbit *after* play-time. This routine makes it less likely that it will eliminate in the wrong places. Also, a hungry rabbit is easily enticed back into its main housing area.

Once the rabbit is neutered, mature, and reliably litter-trained, the routine can be changed. Play sessions can last for hours with the rabbit voluntarily returning to its litter pan whenever necessary to eliminate. For the mature well trained rabbit, it may be advisable to feed it *before* a long, less closely supervised play session. The rabbit with a full stomach may be less likely to chew on household objects. Daily exercise will help minimize obesity, behaviour problems, and osteoporosis (bone loss).

RABBIT TEMPERAMENT

The rabbit's temperament is strongly affected by its sex hormones. Sexually mature female rabbits (as young as several months of age) may become aggressive toward the owners, destructive toward objects in the house, and very territorial, attacking people who try to enter an area. Sexually intact rabbits, whether male or female, may spray urine on various household objects. Therefore, it is advisable to neuter both male and female rabbits before sexual maturity or when any of these behavioural changes occur. There are also medical advantages to neutering of rabbits: prevention of uterine cancer and other diseases in the female and prevention of testicular cancer in the male.

Individual rabbits have clearly discernible personalities ranging from timid to aggressive. A rabbit (even if neutered) may be the dominant member of a group of rabbits housed together and yet may be quite fearful of human beings; the opposite can also be true.

SPECIFIC BEHAVIOUR PROBLEMS

It is important to gather background information in order to evaluate a rabbit behaviour problem. A detailed schedule of the rabbit's routine activities will help when planning behaviour modification strategies. A complete history of the problem may provide clues to any inciting factors. Understanding the relationship of the rabbit to the people and other animals in the home will help in devising solutions to the problem. A thorough physical examination provides information for ruling out a physiological cause of the problem and for deciding whether clinical diagnostic tests are indicated.

Chewing on inappropriate objects

Wires, television remote control buttons, books, furniture, carpet, clothing and wallpaper are among the many household objects that rabbits find particularly appealing. Electrical wires are of special concern because of the possibility of fire and the potential of injury or electrocution of the rabbit.

A rabbit may temporarily become obsessed with something, e.g. playing with the toilet paper (Figure 10.7) or chewing on the furniture. This usually lasts about a week. The owner can try thumping loudly with his or her foot, or spraying the rabbit with water (or air) if it is possible to catch the rabbit in the act. A confident rabbit may give a head shake in response to the owner's thumping or other attempts to correct its behaviour. The head shake seems to be a playful (or defiant) reaction to the correction, and the rabbit may return to the undesirable activity in a short period of time.

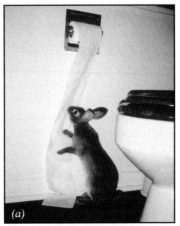

Figure 10.7: Playing with the toilet paper.

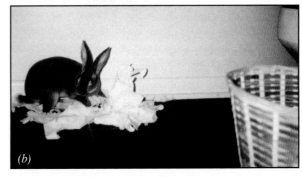

Other than a direct correction for chewing on inappropriate objects, the owner can offer the rabbit something better to chew, like a carrot, a piece of broccoli, or an acceptable toy. Suitable cage toys for a rabbit include junk mail, empty paper towel rolls, sturdy cat toys with bells, small cloth stuffed toys and a children's toy key ring. A game that will distract some rabbits is 'Super Bunny', where the rabbit races around the house with a small towel over its back. Returning the rabbit to its pen for a rest period is another method of interrupting the unwanted chewing behaviour.

By far the easiest way of dealing with inappropriate chewing behaviour is to close the door to certain rooms and to 'rabbit-proof' the rooms of the house where the rabbit will be allowed to play. The owner should place certain valuable items out of the rabbit's reach (remembering that rabbits are natural climbers). Some adjustments can be made, such as scrubbing out the fireplace to allow the rabbit to use that area as a special hiding place (Figure 10.8).

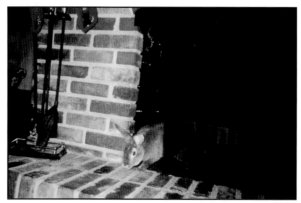

Figure 10.8: Rabbit emerging from the fireplace.

Some rabbits are repelled by such scents as perfumes, cat repellents, and menthol used in ointments for sore muscles. Blankets or large towels can protect 'tantalizing' furniture, and plexiglas sheets and garden aluminium strips can cover portions of walls, floors and baseboards. Electrical wires are the most problematical; however, furniture can be rearranged to hide them. Another way of protecting wires is to cover them with flexible tubing that is not easily chewed by a rabbit. Examples of such tubing are heavy plastic tubing split lengthwise and flexible metal tubing (used for shower hoses). Hardware and home improvement stores sell such items.

The rabbit quickly learns how to open doors within the house unless the doors are securely latched. A rabbit will push on a door or tug on its edge to open it. A computer room (with all the specialized computer cables) is one that an owner might wish to declare 'off limits' to the rabbit.

Inappropriate elimination

If the rabbit is newly acquired, the owner should limit the length of each play session outside the rabbit's pen to 30 minutes. The young rabbit, like a puppy, may be easily distracted by its surroundings. A well established habit of using the litter box in the travelling crate will ease the adjustment to a new home if the owner moves or travels with the rabbit (Figure 10.9).

Inappropriate elimination behaviour in a well adjusted house rabbit is usually limited to sexually intact rabbits, but some rabbits never exhibit this behaviour. A sexually intact rabbit may spray urine on a variety of objects, including the floor, the walls, furniture, other

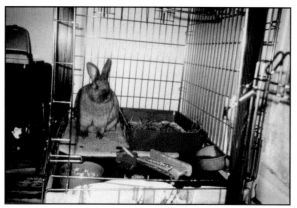

Figure 10.9: Rabbit sitting in a travelling crate.

pets, the owner's bed, the owner, and the owner's friends. Although breeding onset usually does not occur before 4 months in females and 6 months in males, there have been cases of rabbits as young as 3 months spraying their owners. Some sexually intact rabbits defecate throughout the home or the pen.

An intact rabbit, even if more than 1 year of age, usually stops or dramatically decreases this behaviour if surgical neutering is performed. It may take longer for behavioural changes to occur in the female rabbit (months) than in the male rabbit (days to weeks) after neutering.

Inappropriate mating behaviour

The sexually intact male rabbit may attempt to mount other animal species (dogs, cats) or the feet of a human, especially if the person is wearing furry slippers. Prior to the mating attempt, the rabbit generally makes a humming sound while circling the object of his affection. Neutering the rabbit will solve or greatly diminish this problem.

Nesting behaviour

Nesting behaviour is common in the sexually intact adult female rabbit. Characteristics of the nesting behaviour include increased chewing of household objects and protecting her territory. The rabbit may attack people and other animals who come into her area. The area is defined by the rabbit and may include one or more entire rooms of the home. An ovariohysterectomy will eliminate or greatly diminish this behaviour.

Fearful, timid behaviour

In general, rabbits do not like to be picked up, unless they have been handled a great deal when very young. Owners can ease a rabbit's fears by closely analysing and minimizing the situations that seem to elicit fearful reactions. A young child, for example, by moving quickly or by trying to hold the rabbit, may induce panic in a timid rabbit. A parent should supervise child–rabbit interactions carefully and teach the child how to be a friend to the rabbit. A frightened rabbit will stamp its hind feet (a natural warning signal for other rabbits). The rabbit may freeze or run in such a situation. In a frightened rabbit, the nictitating membranes cover part of each eye. When trying to reassure a very fearful young animal, the owner can put the rabbit in a towel-lined small box and pet the animal while watching television. If the owner is patient, most timid rabbits will learn to trust the owner and even to become more confident with strangers and with children.

Aggression toward people

Rabbits, like other animals, have distinct personalities. One dimension of an animal's personality involves the animal's perception of its place in the household hierarchy. Dominance behaviour in rabbits may be manifested toward people as growling, biting, or scratching. This behaviour may occur as the rabbit reaches puberty. It is somewhat more common in female rabbits than in male rabbits. Surgical neutering can decrease, but not necessarily eliminate, aggressive behaviour.

When a rabbit acts aggressively toward its owner, the person should notice the circumstances in which the behaviour occurred. A lively rabbit who is in the midst of dashing about the house may react aggressively if the owner interrupts this playfulness and tries to pet it. However, if aggression toward the owner is completely spontaneous, the owner should discourage this behaviour by saying 'eek' or 'ow', or by spraying the rabbit with water.

A rabbit may also exhibit territorial aggression while being lifted out of a cage. If this occurs, the owner should throw a towel over it before removing it from its cage. A rabbit may also show signs of aggression when a person enters its room or pen. The owner can modify this behaviour by sitting down in the play area (with arms and legs well covered with heavy clothing or blankets). A box or a hay bale between the rabbit and the person provides a partial barrier. A variety of items for safe chewing should be placed in the enclosure. The owner should read a book and pretend to ignore the rabbit. If the rabbit approaches, the owner can offer some treats.

The stages in a rabbit's anger have been accurately described in detail by Bill Markwick, writing on the PetBunny Internet list. Initially, the rabbit holds its ears tightly to its back. In the second stage, the rabbit punches the person with its front paws. This is harmless, but startling! If its anger escalates, the rabbit may give a warning by butting against the person with its mouth held stiffly open so that the surface of the incisors makes contact with the person. Ultimately, the angry rabbit may bite the person.

Misdirected rabbit bites to a person can occur if the person is trying to separate two rabbits who are fighting. Fighting rabbits should be separated with brooms or other objects to prevent such injuries.

Aggression toward other rabbits

Dominance behaviour is probably the cause of aggression toward other rabbits. This behaviour is not eliminated by surgical neutering. As with other household pets (e.g. dogs and cats), creating compatible groups of rabbits can be a challenge. The section of this chapter on General Training Tips offers some suggestions for introducing rabbits to each other. Even apparently well bonded rabbits who have lived together for months or years may injure each other. Bite wounds needing veterinary attention are commonly found on the face or hind quarters.

Unfortunately, one rabbit may become a social outcast in groups of three or more rabbits. This has been observed both in nature and in domestic situations. Provided that the loner rabbit observes the rules of minimum distance, it may be safe from attack, but such a rabbit may lose condition or become excessively fearful.

Aggression toward other animals

The rabbit may dominate other household pets, including cats and even large dogs. Such situations must be monitored for the rabbit's protection. A warning from a dog could be fatal to the rabbit. Generally, a rabbit can live peacefully with dogs and cats, but these animals should not be left together while the owner is absent. A rabbit is as mischievous as a small child and may provoke a dog into taking aggressive or defensive action.

CONCLUSION

Rabbit behaviour is very different from dog and cat behaviour. An owner who understands dominance behaviour in rabbits, for example, will not be surprised that the animal lying quietly to be petted will suddenly chew on the furniture. Rabbits are obviously endearing pets, because owners love them despite some of their natural behaviours that can wreak havoc in a household. Examples of rabbit owners' devotion can be found using a computer to access the World Wide Web sites dedicated to pet rabbits. The *100 Question ToughBun Purity Test* is a hilarious listing of annoying rabbit behaviours, and the *100 Question Slave Purity Test* refers to owners as 'bunny slaves'. Books on rabbit care and letters to the editor of house rabbit journals also contain tributes to rabbits.

The rabbit is a delightful pet: clean, lively, affectionate, and curious. Its normal nap time is during the day, when most owners are at work or school. Outdoor exercise is not necessary for the rabbit so it is an easy animal to maintain in a flat. Shaping a rabbit's behaviour to live in a house with people will yield a joyful companionship for both parties to the human–rabbit bond.

REFERENCES AND FURTHER READING

Harriman M (1991) *House Rabbit Handbook: How to Live with an Urban Rabbit* (revised edition). Drollery Press, Alameda, California
House Rabbit Journal (1992–present), published quarterly, House Rabbit Society, Alameda, California
Hunter S (1991) *Hop To It: A Guide to Training Your Pet Rabbit.* Barron's Educational Series Inc., Hauppauge, New York
Lockley RM (1974) *The Private Life of the Rabbit.* Macmillan Publishing Co., New York
Okerman L (1994) *Diseases of Domestic Rabbits, 2nd edn.* Blackwell, Oxford
PetBunny Internet List: LISTSERV@LSV.UKY.EDU Send message: SUBscribe PETBUNNY
Rabbiting On (1997–present), published quarterly, British Houserabbit Association, Newcastle-upon-Tyne World Wide Web address: http://www.houserabbit.co.uk
Roberts M (1996) *The Man Who Listens to Horses.* Random House, New York

The 100 Question Toughbun Purity Test, http://www.planetx.org/~bunny/toughbun.html
The 100 Question Slave Purity Test, http://www.planetx.org/~bunny/purity.html
Turner RJ, Held SD, Hirst JE, Billinghurst G and Wootton RJ (1997) An immunological assessment of group-housed rabbits. *Laboratory Animals* **31**, 362–372
Wegler M (1989) *Rabbits: How to Take Care of Them and Understand Them.* Barron's Educational Series Inc., Hauppauge, New York

AUTHOR'S ACKNOWLEDGEMENT

Dr Christine Williams and Dr Richard Walshaw patiently read several drafts of this chapter and reminded me to be thorough when writing it. A special thank you is extended to Richard and Patty Walshaw for allowing their photographs to be used in this book. Finally, I am indebted to the lessons I have received over the past 30 years from my lovable house rabbits: Thumper, Max, Monroe, Butterscotch, and Raymond.

CHAPTER ELEVEN

Therapeutics

Timothy H. Morris

INTRODUCTION

The importance of therapeutics

There are few texts devoted to pet rabbit medicine and surgery, and within them therapeutics is rarely considered separately. There are good reasons for this, as the study of pet rabbit therapeutics is in its infancy; however, it is important to lay a sound scientific basis for veterinary treatment of this increasingly common pet. Therapeutics is the study of drug treatment, including selection, administration, formulation and practical use. It is important to understand that the tables of drug dosages commonly found in texts and formularies are an example of the more limited, but complementary, discipline of posology, which confines itself to drug dosage.

This chapter will focus on prescribing legislation, physiological and pharmacokinetic factors, the background to extrapolating doses between species, and what is known about specific drugs in the rabbit.

Finding drug dosages

Ultimately, rational drug treatment does involve defining the dosage, so the sources of this information must be clear. Within the other chapters of this book drug dosages are given in the text, and in the references cited. Formularies are also available. The *BSAVA Small Animal Formulary* (Tennant, 1999) is a useful and well presented starting point for rabbit drug doses but, in common with the majority of formularies, the specific source of many doses are either not given or are obtained from other compilations or review articles. One exception is the *Formulary for Laboratory Animals* (Hawk and Leary, 1999) which gives a reference for every dosage and attempts to cite specific studies whenever possible. A summary of a selection of drug dosages is given in Figure 11.1, but clinicians are advised to read this chapter first to enable safe and efficacious drug use.

DRUG	DOSE
Antifungal agent	
Griseofulvin	25 mg/kg; p.o. q24h, or divided q12h for 28–40 days
Antiparasitic agents	
Amprolium 9.6% solution	1 ml/7 kg; p.o. q24h for 5 days, or 0.5 ml/500 ml drinking water for 10 days
Fenbendazole	20 mg/kg q24h for 5 days; p.o.
Ivermectin	200–400 µg/kg; p.o., s.c.; repeat in 8–10 days
Piperazine adipate	0.5 g/kg q24h for 2 days; p.o.
Piperazine citrate	100 mg/kg q24h for 2 days; p.o.
Praziquantel	5–10 mg/kg; p.o., s.c., i.m; repeat in 10 days
Sulphadimethoxine	25–50 mg/kg q24h, or 50 mg/kg loading dose followed by 25mg/kg q24h for 9 days; p.o.
Sulphaquinoxaline	1 mg/ml drinking water
Thiabendazole	100–200mg/kg p.o. once

Figure 11.1: Formulary for rabbits. Drug dose rates compiled from a variety of sources (Hawke and Leary, 1995; Johnson-Delaney, 1996; Laber Laird et al., 1996; Hillyer and Quesenberry, 1997; Flecknell, 1998) and from rates quoted by authors in this Manual. In most instances, dose rates have been established by clinical experience, and few agents have been adequately evaluated in rabbits. It is therefore advisable to exercise caution when treating rabbits, and to monitor the effects of therapy carefully. Where dose rates have been quoted as a total dose per rabbit, it is assumed that this refers to an average 4 kg animal, however dose rates have not been translated into mg/kg, to avoid giving a false impression of precision. Refer to text for further information on estimation of dose rates, and of the particular caution needed when using antibiotics. ▶

DRUG	DOSE
Antibiotics	
Amikacin	8–16 mg/kg total dose*; divided q8–24h; s.c., i.m., i.v.
Cephalexin	15 mg/kg s.c. twice daily
Chloramphenicol	50 mg/kg p.o. once daily 15 mg/kg i.m. twice daily
Chlortetracycline	1 g/l drinking water; 50 mg/kg q12h; p.o.
Ciprofloxacin	5–15 mg/kg q12h; p.o.
Clopidol	200 g/tonne feed
Dimetridazole	0.2 mg/ml drinking water
Doxycycline	2.5 mg/kg q12h; p.o.
Enrofloxacin	5–15 mg/kg q12h; p.o, s.c, i.m.
Gentamicin	5–8 mg/kg total dose*; divided q8–24h; s.c., i.m, i.v.
Griseofulvin	25 mg/kg p.o. once daily for 4 weeks
Metronidazole	20 mg/kg q12h; p.o. for 3–5 days
Neomycin	30 mg/kg q12h; p.o.
Oxytetracycline	50 mg/kg q12h; p.o; 15 mg/kg q24h; s.c., i.m.
Penicillin G procaine	20,000–60,000 IU/kg q24h; s.c., i.m.
Penicillin G benzathine and penicillin G procaine	47,000–84,000 IU/kg once per wk; s.c., i.m. (for *Treponema cuniculi* infection)
Robenidine	50–66 g/tonne feed
Streptomycin	50 mg/kg i.m. once daily
Sulphadiazine/trimethoprim	48 mg/kg s.c. once daily
Sulphadimidine	100–233 mg/l drinking water
Sulphamethazine	1–5 mg/ml drinking water
Sulphamethoxazole/trimethoprim	15–30 mg/kg q12h; p.o.
Tetracycline	50 mg/kg q8–12h; p.o.
Tylosin	10 mg/kg q12h; p.o, s.c., i.m.
Other agents	
Calcium gluconate	5–10 ml of 10% soln i.v. per adult rabbit
Cholestyramine resin	2 g p.o. per adult rabbit/day (equivalent of 4 g of 'Questran'/day)
Cisapride	0.5 mg/kg q8–24h, p.o.
Dexamethasone	2–4 mg/kg s.c. or i.v. (as an adjunct to the management of shock), 0.2 mg/kg s.c. or i.m. as an anti-inflammatory
Furosemide	0.3–2 mg/kg q12h p.o., s.c., i.m., i.v.
Hydrocortisone	10 mg/kg i.m., i.v.
Lasalocid	120 ppm added to feed
Metoclopramide	0.5 mg/kg q8h, s.c.
Oxytocin	1–2 units i.m., s.c. per adult rabbit
Prednisolone	0.5–2 mg/kg p.o., i.m., s.c.
Simethicone	20–40 mg p.o. per adult rabbit, q4–6h

*Figure 11.1 continued: Formulary for rabbits. Drug dose rates compiled from a variety of sources (Hawke and Leary, 1995; Johnson-Delaney, 1996; Laber Laird et al., 1996; Hillyer and Quesenberry, 1997; Flecknell, 1998) and from rates quoted by authors in this Manual. In most instances, dose rates have been established by clinical experience, and few agents have been adequately evaluated in rabbits. It is therefore advisable to exercise caution when treating rabbits, and to monitor the effects of therapy carefully. *Where dose rates have been quoted as a total dose per rabbit, it is assumed that this refers to an average 4 kg animal, however dose rates have not been translated into mg/kg, to avoid giving a false impression of precision. Refer to text for further information on estimation of dose rates, and of the particular caution needed when using antibiotics.*

How are dosages established?

In pet rabbits, therapeutic drug dosages are derived from four broad sources:

- Rabbits have been used in meat production and as laboratory animals for many years. Therapies discovered from empirical use and in specific studies have been transferred to pet rabbits. Whilst this source remains important, the different husbandry, different animal strains, and differing perspectives of pet and commercial rabbit care do limit applicability
- Practitioners have empirically developed effective treatment regimes for pet rabbits and this information has been disseminated formally through publications and presentations, and informally through meetings and the Internet
- In many of the situations above, dosages are extrapolated from dose rates for other species
- There have been a relatively small number of studies where treatment regimes have been tested and evaluated in clinical trials, and then disseminated to practitioners.

How therapeutics can help in rational treatment

The quantitative science of pharmacokinetics provides the bridge between the therapeutic window and the required dosage regime (Riviere, 1995). A drug's pharmacokinetics depends on the interrelationship between the drug and the animal's physiology and anatomy. The drug's physicochemical properties are defined both by the active drug itself but also, more importantly, by the formulation of the drug.

The animal's anatomy and physiology will affect the absorption of drugs and often affect routes of administration, influence the distribution of drugs, dictate their metabolism and affect drug excretion. All these factors come together when attempting to develop the most appropriate dosage to get the optimum amount of drug to the required site of action, and to limit and understand its side effects. For more details, a useful practitioner-orientated overview of the theory and practice of pharmacokinetics in veterinary medicine has been published recently (Martinez, 1998a,b,c,d,e).

LEGISLATION AFFECTING PRESCRIBING FOR PET RABBITS

For the majority of animals seen by veterinary surgeons, approved drugs are available. This means their safety and efficacy is assessed and, most usefully, that they are supplied with a data sheet with details of dose rate and frequency, routes of administration, safety and, if applicable, withdrawal periods. Few drugs are approved for rabbits; these are limited to vaccines, a small number of antimicrobials and parasiticides, and a few miscellaneous drugs such as anaesthetics (Hayhow, 1998).

Thus, in most cases, the veterinary surgeon will be prescribing an unapproved drug. In most countries there are specific rules to allow this. For example, in the European Union, the phrase 'an animal or a small number of animals on a particular holding' also covers pets, and should be interpreted more flexibly for minor or exotic animal species which do not produce food (European Commission, 1990). Similarly, in the USA the Food and Drug Administration has issued a final rule to allow veterinarians to prescribe extralabel uses of certain approved animal drugs and approved human drugs for animals (Federal Register, 1996). Elsewhere, at the very least, there is usually some understanding that flexibility in prescribing be considered in the interests of animal welfare.

Specifically in the UK, guidelines provided by the Veterinary Medicines Directorate (VMD, 1995) appear to exclude pet rabbits from the strict controls of the 'prescribing cascade'.

It is important for veterinary surgeons to be fully aware of the relevant legislation and/or practices in the country where they are working and to recognize that any flexibility would be confined to pet rabbits. It is important to note that drugs given to laboratory rabbits may affect the research study in which these animals are being used (Morris, 1995) and especially note that rules for rabbits reared for meat production would be much more stringent (VMD, 1995; Federal Register, 1996).

Another consideration in the choice of drug is its preparation or formulation. While some flexibility in use of human preparations may be introduced by the legislation described above, it should be recognized that human formulations are designed for use in a different environment; for example, oily injectable and depot preparations are more common in veterinary practice but not well accepted in human medicine, where aqueous injectable preparations are more common. These latter preparations have a much shorter duration of action. Formulation differences between different brands, which use different salt forms, solvents and excipients, affect therapeutics of a particular product by altering bioavailability (the rate and extent of absorption of the same drug in the same dosage form).

Bioinequivalence (defined as differences in bioavailability between the same drug dosage form) has been clearly shown in other species (Morris, 1995). A more practical advantage of using veterinary preparations is that the drug companies' veterinary advisors may well have on file efficacy and safety data in rabbits, either from reported use, or from basic pharmacokinetic and toxicity studies. Access to this information can be important in limiting liability when prescribing unapproved drugs.

ABSORPTION, DISTRIBUTION, METABOLISM AND EXCRETION OF DRUGS

Absorption

The absorption of a drug depends on its physicochemical properties, its formulation and its route of administration. The formulation of a commercial preparation will be optimized for the physicochemical properties of the active drug, for the species for which it is intended. Many drugs may not be formulated optimally for the physiological and anatomical peculiarities of the rabbit.

Drugs given orally to rabbits pass through the mouth, where the herbivorous diet dictates the need for prolonged mastication, and where amylase is present in the saliva. This contrasts with the dog and cat, where food is swallowed more rapidly, and amylase is not present. Drug absorption from the buccal cavity, with subsequent rapid distribution and avoidance of hepatic metabolism, could be more prominent in the rabbit compared to carnivores. As starch is commonly used as an excipient in oral preparations, product dissolution may be more rapid in the amylase-rich rabbit saliva.

Rabbits are tolerant of bitter tastes but such preparations (e.g. some oral fluoroquinolone preparations) may be difficult for owners to administer for long periods. As rabbits prefer sweet tastes, flavouring such as fruit juices can be used to enhance acceptance.

Once a drug has entered the stomach, its subsequent passage to the intestinal tract depends on gastric emptying, which is dependent on the time of day; rabbits mainly feed at night and early morning. The rabbit's stomach is very acid, pH 1–2, compared to 3–4 in the dog and cat (Rozman, 1988). The pK_a of a drug affects its ionization, and thus its absorption, as generally only un-ionized drugs will be absorbed (Martinez, 1998c).

The rabbit is adapted to a fibrous plant-based diet, and liquids and particulates are handled differently. Gastric emptying time for fluids is about 1.3 hours, and for particulates 12 hours, compared to 1.5 hours for both in the dog (Kararli, 1995). The small intestine of the rabbit is relatively short, about 12% of the total volume of the gastrointestinal tract, compared to 22% in the dog, and with a poorer blood supply. The rabbit's large intestine is large: the caecum has about 40% of the capacity of the gastrointestinal tract (Kararli, 1995). Thus, orally administered drugs may be relatively poorly absorbed, or absorbed over a longer period due to trapping in the caecum.

The differential passage rates of fluid and fibre are reflected in the percentage of fluid and particulate markers excreted in the faeces: 24 hours after intragastric administration, 25% of a fluid marker was excreted compared to 54% of a particulate marker (the respective figures for the dog were 55% and 40%).

This difference is emphasized by data from experimental intracaecal administration, where 30% of fluid markers were excreted compared to 96% of particulate markers (Kararli, 1995). One interpretation of this information is that fluid formulations will be retained longer, whereas particulate formulations, or, more likely, drugs that bind to particulate matter, will be excreted more quickly. Caecotrophy (eating caecal matter) is integral to digestion in rabbits (see Chapter 5) and this has the potential to recycle drugs further.

The widely held paradigm that absorption of drugs is greater from intramuscular injection than from subcutaneous injection may not be correct. Work in calves and dogs showed that subcutaneous absorption was similar to intramuscular absorption (Morris, 1995). Practical implications in rabbits stem from concerns on the volumes that are safe and humane to inject. Recommended maximal volumes for intramuscular injections in the rabbit are 0.3–1.0 ml (Hawk and Leary, 1999) but extrapolation of this dose volume from a 3.5 kg rabbit to a 70 kg man gives a dose volume of 6–20 ml, emphasizing the welfare concerns. Compounding this concern is the fact that, as explained in the later part of this chapter (see also Figure 11.4), the higher metabolic rates of rabbits compared to larger species mean that relatively higher dose rates are required.

As veterinary preparations are formulated for larger species, the dose volumes required for rabbits may be quite high. For example, a 50 mg/ml oxytetracycline injection preparation, given at a dose rate of 15 mg/kg, gives a dose volume of over 1 ml for a 3.5 kg rabbit. Subcutaneous injection is therefore a good alternative to consider in the rabbit, although one concern would stem from the tendency towards obesity, leading to the possibility that injections may be made into fat deposits.

Some other anatomical features may influence drug absorption. The path of the nasolacrimal duct is not straight (Marini et al., 1996); in addition, in rabbits with chronic dental disease, inflammation of the tooth root may cause this to become the point of blockage. This may affect absorption of drugs instilled into the palpebral opening.

The glottis of the rabbit is small and covered by the tongue. If oxygen therapy or nebulization is used in a collapsed rabbit, then the tongue should be pulled forward to uncover the glottis. Nebulization can also be used to deliver drugs via the nostrils. Nasogastric intubation is also feasible in the rabbit, but the nostrils, being well equipped with touch cells, are very sensitive, so the use of topical local anaesthetics should be considered.

Compared with other small mammal pets, rabbits have large ears: on average, 12% of the body surface area. The marginal ear vein makes intravenous injections, using catheters or butterfly needles, straightforward in all but the dwarf breeds, which have smaller ears. Chronic venous access via this vein is possible (Melich, 1990).

Distribution

Once absorbed, drugs are distributed around the body, decreasing their concentration. Many drugs are protein-bound. Serum proteins in the rabbit are not significantly different from those of other species, but binding at other sites may be different. The bony skeleton comprises only about 8% of bodyweight in the rabbit, compared to about 13% in the cat. Drugs that are sequestered in bone, such as tetracyclines, therefore have a smaller reservoir. Obesity is common in pet rabbits, and highly lipid-soluble drugs, e.g. thiopentone, propranolol and organophosphates, probably accumulate to a greater extent, and persist longer (Wyss *et al.*, 1982).

Drug distribution can be described in terms of discrete body compartments. The large caecum can be considered as a significant compartment for distribution in the rabbit. As in ruminants, it should be considered a reservoir for absorption, especially for lipid-soluble bases (Martinez, 1986b) but also, because of significant bile production and caecotrophy, a compartment for distribution. The increased total volume of distribution will increase the half-life of drugs persisting in the rabbit caecum. Total body water is also relatively higher in rabbits (0.72 l/kg, compared to 0.60 l/kg in dogs and man, and 0.67 l/kg in rats (Lave *et al.*, 1999) and this also affects drug distribution (Davies and Morris, 1993).

The volume of distribution, protein binding and other characteristics, such as partition coefficient of a drug in some species, may be available from the drug manufacturer. A list of these parameters for 125 clinically useful drugs has been published, although some parameters are applicable only in humans (Ritschel and Hammer, 1980).

Metabolism

Differences in the way drugs are biotransformed are the best documented causes for differences in drug disposition. For example, the research on, and subsequent approval of, many drugs in the cat has led to a greater understanding of how the metabolic peculiarities in that species affect therapy (Evans, 1985). However, in the rabbit, biotransformation is relatively poorly understood, compared to other small mammal pets such as rats and mice. Whereas rats and mice are used

as laboratory animals for the carcinogenicity testing of medicines, as the carcinogenic process is proportional to lifespan, animals selected as models are those that have a lifespan of 2–3 years, and so this excludes the longer-lived rabbit.

The main reason for interspecies variation in metabolism is that there are differences in the rates and types of enzymatic control of Phase I & II reactions that effect biotransformation.

Phase I

Phase I reactions – oxidation, reduction or hydrolysis – change the drug (usually inactivating it, although sometimes an inactive precursor becomes the active form).

Phase II

Phase II reactions conjugate the product with compounds derived from carbohydrates and amino acids, e.g. glucuronic acid, glycine, methionine and sulphates, to produce a strong acid that is typically readily excreted in the bile or urine.

The principal site for these enzymes is the liver, but they are also found in the cells of the kidney, lung, olfactory membranes and intestine. In their microsomes the principal enzyme is cytochrome P-450. In the rabbit, at least eight P-450 isoenzymes have been identified in the liver, seven in olfactory microsomes and at least two in the lungs; variations in activity and type of reaction have been reported (Wolf *et al.*, 1979; Anderson and Henk, 1994). Generally, rabbit liver microsomal activity ranges from that similar to the rat, to 10 times less than this; and in a range from a rate similar to, to one approximately 5 times greater than that of the dog or cat (Walker, 1978). Much of this difference is related to metabolic rates, which are higher in smaller animals (see discussion below on metabolic scaling), thus there is little species peculiarity in the rate of microsomal activity in the rabbit.

However, there are clear peculiarities in the type of reaction in the rabbit. These examples are drawn from studies on human drug safety assessment, although some extrapolations can be made from one drug to another; for example, paracetamol is an aniline derivative (Figure 11.2). As well as these differences, there are some examples of differences between individuals;

Drug	Phase I reactions	Phase II reactions
Coumarin	Hydroxylation in man Reduction in rats Both hydroxylation and reduction in rabbits	*N*-acetylglucosamine: an uncommon conjugate used by rabbits
Amphetamines	Hydroxylation in rats Oxidation in guinea-pigs and rabbits	Intestinal uridine diphosphate glycostransferase activity higher in rabbits than in rats
Aniline	*p*-Hydroxylation in rodents and rabbits *o*-Hydroxylation in dogs and cats	

Figure 11.2: *Example of species differences in drug biotransformation. Data from Smith (1974); Anderson and Henk (1994); Lin (1998); Rozman (1998).*

for example, there are fast and slow acetylator rabbits (Anderson and Henk, 1994), variable levels of atropine esterase (Olson *et al.,* 1993), and variations in the expression of P-450 between individual rabbits, irrespective of strain (Johnson and Griffin, 1985).

It is therefore probable that the metabolism of some commonly used therapeutic drugs will be different in the rabbit, due to peculiarities in the types and balance of Phase I and Phase II reactions. However, specific knowledge of how this affects most medicinal drug therapy is quite unknown at this time. Clinicians should, therefore, be alert to the possibility of these peculiarities producing unexpected responses after drugs that are safely used in other species are used in the rabbit.

Excretion

The most important route of excretion is via the kidney, with the second most important route via the faeces. Biotransformed drugs may arrive at the kidney differently, or after resorption from the gut after biliary excretion. The balance of excretion is often determined by whether the predominant metabolism is Phase I or II. For example, rabbits metabolize griseofulvin mainly via a Phase I reaction, thus excreting it mainly via the urine, while rats metabolize griscofulvin via Phase II reactions to a much greater extent, and thus excrete it mostly in bile (Rozman,1988).

The rabbit kidney has both morphological and functional peculiarities. The number of glomeruli active at any one time can vary and increased hydration, leading to up to a 16-fold increase in diuresis, is mediated not by increased glomerular filtration rate but by activation of more glomeruli. Thus, for those drugs that are well absorbed and undergo minimal biotransformation, and so are excreted directly by glomerular filtration (e.g. furosemide), the state of hydration can very rapidly change excretion rates in the rabbit. The clinical impact of the other physiological peculiarities of the rabbit kidney on medicinal drug excretion is as yet unclear; for example, relatively inefficient resorption of bicarbonate, lack of carbonic hydrase in the thick ascending tubules of the kidney and enzymatic differences in handling ammonia (Brewer and Cruise, 1994).

Bile flow in the rabbit is unusually high: up to 130 ml/kg/day compared to 19–36 ml/kg/day in the dog and 48–92 ml/kg/day in the rat, although this may not necessarily correlate with biliary excretion of drugs (Lin, 1998). Bacterial hydrolysis of glucuronide conjugates excreted in bile into the gut play a major role in enterohepatic drug circulation. There is evidence that this activity is less in the rabbit than in rodents (Kararli, 1995), possibly leading to higher faecal excretion of conjugated compounds in rabbits compared to rodents, and the possibility that metabolites with the potential for caecal dysbiosis are more likely to be delivered to the large rabbit caecum.

In conclusion, there are considerable anatomical and physiological peculiarities in the rabbit with potential to affect drug absorption, distribution, metabolism and excretion, and limited evidence from studies on drugs intended for man that these peculiarities can significantly affect medicinal drug therapeutics. As there is almost no practical information at the moment to guide the clinician in rationale and safe therapy, it is especially important to adopt a cautious appproach to therapeutics in the rabbit.

USING KNOWLEDGE OF DRUG DOSES FROM OTHER SPECIES TO TREAT RABBITS

Background to interspecies scaling

It is known that many anatomical and physiological factors are mathematical functions of bodyweight; it has been found that, in species spanning a wide weight range, for over a hundred diverse biological parameters the relation is linear to body weight. The equation that describes this relationship is:

$$\log P = \log (a + b) \times \log W$$

where P is the parameter of interest, W the bodyweight, a the intercept fixing P when bodyweight equals 1 kg, and b the exponent (the slope of the line).

This can be simplified to:

$$P = aW^b$$

The exponent (slope) varies with the parameter; the exponent for volumes of organs (heart, lung, etc.) is about 1, because relative to each other and to the body as a whole they are indispensable, thus they increase in proportion directly to increased size. The skeleton, in contrast, is required to be stronger in larger animals and thus the exponent is greater than 1.

When considering drug dosage, the principal size-dependent species difference is metabolic rate, where the exponent is 0.75. If it is assumed that anatomical features and biochemical reactions are similar within the same Class (e.g. mammals, reptiles), then there are consequences as organisms increase in size. The body surface area to bodyweight ratio falls as animals get larger, and thus the ability to lose heat also falls. Metabolic processes are optimized for a particular temperature. Evolutionary pressure, with increasing size, is to choose between controlling this inability to lose heat by a fundamental change in metabolic processes, or to reduce metabolic rate. The evolved adaptation to reduce metabolic rate explains the observations that in species spanning a wide weight range, physiological parameters, such as oxygen consumption, ventilation rate, renal clearance and nitrogen output only correlate linearly when plotted across bodyweight on a log:log scale with an exponent of about 0.75.

The consequences are clear. As body size increases, these physiological parameters are relatively reduced; for example, 1 g of shrew tissue has a metabolic rate 1000 times greater than 1 g of blue whale tissue. The duration of processes such as cardiac cycle, lifespan and drug half-life, when plotted against bodyweight also correlate linearly when a log:log scale is used, with the exponent being 0.25.

This also means that drugs are exposed to the liver and kidneys more quickly and more frequently. As body size increases, the duration of processes increases; for example, compare the short lifespan of the shrew and the long lifespan of the blue whale.

The underlying basis for allometric scaling has in the past been understood on a somewhat empirical basis. Recently it has been suggested to be based on the evolutionary pressure to maximize metabolic capacity by use of distribution networks to distribute resource and remove waste in an organism (West *et al.*, 1999; Morris, 2000).

Using scaling to predict drug doses across species

Differences between species relative to drugs can be size-independent or size-dependent. Differences in biotransformation are independent of size. A major source of error in extrapolation of dose across species when this is done on a mg/kg basis is that it fails to take into account the size-dependent effect of differences in metabolic rate on drug pharmacokinetics.

How can metabolic rate be taken into consideration? Allometry is the study of size and its consequences, concentrating on those scaling factors related to the influence of size on metabolism, excluding size-independent factors such as different metabolic routes. The basic allometric principle is expressed in the equation $P = aW^b$ described above, and has been used to extrapolate pharmacokinetic parameters across a wide range of species. Variable applicability has been noted; recently in a study when 44 compounds were assessed, only 11 showed significant allometric correlations (many of these were antibiotics), and 13 showed less robust correlation (Riviere *et al.*, 1997).

The principal reason for this lack of universal applicability is that allometry deals only with size; it does not address the important metabolic differences between species, as discussed above and illustrated in Figure 11.2. As well as the qualitative differences between species, described above in general, those drugs with hepatic metabolism (especially those with low extraction), rather than renal clearance, those drugs where protein binding varies between species, and those drugs that do not have first-order pharmacokinetics are less applicable to allometric scaling. The accuracy of allometric scaling for compounds with hepatic metabolism has been improved by incorporating data from *in vitro* studies.

What factors should be considered by the clinician when using a dosage in rabbits that has been obtained from another species? If the information suggests that metabolic differences will not confound the estimation, it is prudent to calculate drug dosages between species of widely varying bodyweights with a consideration of metabolic rate: i.e. calculations based on mg/kg dose may be less accurate than those based on $mg/kg^{0.75}$. This method is illustrated in Figures 11.3 and 11.4. A computer spreadsheet can be used for these calculations; one is used in a commercially available electronic formulary (Vetbase, Hajeka Informatie & Advies, Graafschap 7, 3524 TL Utrecht, The Netherlands, http://vetinfo.demon.nl).

Dose frequency will increase if a dose frequency in a large species is converted to a dose frequency for a rabbit. In some cases it may be best to alter the dose, but in others it may be better to alter the dose frequency or (for example, if dose frequency or dose volume is too high) to compromise, by estimation, between both changes. It is also important to note that if a drug is formulated for a large species the dose volume will be relatively much larger when this formulation is used in a smaller species, and this may preclude some routes of administration in the rabbit. A fuller explanation of drug dose extrapolation using allometry is found in Morris (1999).

USE OF SPECIFIC DRUG GROUPS IN THE RABBIT

Antibiotics

Toxicity
This is adapted from a more comprehensive article, (Morris, 1995), which gives additional references and greater detail. Clinicians treating rabbits should be aware of the significant potential for antibiotic toxicity in the rabbit. The single most important mechanism of antibiotic toxicity in rabbits is the secondary effects caused by disruption of the normal enteric flora, in particular the effects of toxins produced by *Clostridium perfringens* and *Clostridium spiriforme*. A wide range of antibiotics have been reported as toxic via this mechanism in the rabbit (Figure 11.5).

Lincomycin and clindamycin are particularly dangerous; the toxicity of erythromycin, spectinomycin and minocycline is relatively milder; the situation with penicillins and cephalosporins is less clear.

Ampicillin has been shown to cause serious enteritis with mortality in several studies. Penicillin is acutely toxic, but where penicillin has been claimed to contribute to enteritis, other antibiotics that cause enteritis have also been fed. Indications that penicillin and cephalexin have less potential to cause enteritis than ampicillin come from quantitative faecal bacteriological studies where the antibiotic-induced depression in lactobacilli numbers, and the rise in coliform bacteria and clostridial numbers is less with penicillin and cephalexin than with ampicillin.

1	**Convert reference drug dosage into total dosage and interval format**

Control animal species   _____

Bodyweight of control species (W_{cont})   _____ kg

Dosage rate of control species (rate$_{cont}$)   _____ mg/kg

Route: orally, s.c., i.m., i.v.   _____

Frequency: _____ times/day

Treatment dosage$_{cont}$ = (W_{cont} x rate$_{cont}$) =   _____ mg

Dosing interval$_{cont}$ = 24 hours/frequency =   _____ hours

2	**Calculate parameters that express metabolic size (MEC) and metabolic rate (SMEC) in a format that can be used to compare animals of very different body sizes, using allometric scaling to compare dose quantity** (*use a calculator where necessary*):

Minimum energy cost of the control species (MEC_{cont}) = k ($W^{0.75}$)

Specific minimum energy cost of the control species ($SMEC_{cont}$) = k ($W^{-0.25}$)

where W = bodyweight in kg.

k factors: reptiles = 10 (at 37 °C ambient temperature); passerine birds = 129; non-passerine birds = 78; marsupials = 49; placental mammals = 70.

It is preferable only to scale *within* groups.

3	**Calculate the dosage and interval in terms that can be used for conversion between species, using the data from 1 and 2 above:**

MEC dose = Treatment dosage$_{cont}$ /MEC_{cont} =   _____ mg/kg

SMEC interval = $SMEC_{cont}$ x Dosing interval$_{cont}$ =   _____ hours

4	**Use the MEC dosage and SMEC interval for the drug to derive an allometrically scaled dosage for subject animal species with a very different bodyweight:**

Species of subject animal   _____

Bodyweight of subject animal (W_{subj})   _____ kg

Minimum energy cost of subject animal (MEC_{subj}) = k ($W^{0.75}$)   _____

Specific minimum energy cost of subject animal ($SMEC_{subj}$) = $k(W^{-0.25}$)   _____

Treatment dosage for the subject animal = MEC dosage x MEC_{subj} =   _____ mg

mg/kg dosage = treatment dosage/subject weight =   _____ mg/kg

Treatment interval for the subject animal = SMEC interval/$SMEC_{subj}$ =   _____ hours

Frequency (24 hours/interval) =   _____

Figure 11.3: Allometric dosage and interval scaling worksheet. Adapted from Morris (1999) and developed from a worksheet produced by Charles Sedgwick and modified by Karen Timm, Oregon State University.

1	**Convert reference drug dosage into total dosage and interval format**	
Control animal species	Cow	
Bodyweight of control species (W_{cont})	500	kg
Dosage rate of control species ($rate_{cont}$)	10	mg/kg
Route: orally, s.c., i.m., i.v.		
Frequency:	one	times/day
Treatment dosage$_{cont}$ = (W_{cont} x rate$_{cont}$) =	5000	mg
Dosing interval$_{cont}$ = 24 hours/frequency =	24	hours

2	**Calculate MEC and SMEC:**

Minimum energy cost of the control species (MEC_{cont}) = $k\,(W^{0.75})$ = 7402

Specific minimum energy cost of the control species ($SMEC_{cont}$) = $k\,(W^{-0.25})$ = 14.8

where W = bodyweight in kg.

k factor: placental mammals = 70.

3	**Calculate the dosage and interval:**	
MEC dose = Treatment dosage $_{cont}$/MEC_{cont} =	0.675	mg/kg
SMEC interval = $SMEC_{cont}$ x Dosing interval$_{cont}$ =	355	hours

4	**Derive an allometrically scaled dosage:**	
Species of subject animal	Rabbit	
Bodyweight of subject animal (W_{subj})	3.5	kg

Minimum energy cost of subject animal (MEC_{subj}) = $k\,(W^{0.75})$ = 179

Specific minimum energy cost of subject animal ($SMEC_{subj}$) = $k(W^{-0.25})$ = 51

Treatment dosage for the subject animal = MEC dosage x MEC_{subj} =	121	mg
mg/kg dosage = treatment dosage/subject weight =	34.6	mg/kg
Treatment interval for the subject animal = SMEC interval/$SMEC_{subj}$ =	6.94	hours
Frequency (24 hours/interval) =	3 times a day	

Either the relative dosage needs to be increased from 10 mg/kg in the cow to 35 mg/kg in the rabbit, or the cow dosage needs to be given 3 times a day to the rabbit. Note also that the dose volume, using a 100 mg/ml presentation, is 1.2 ml/rabbit (0.35 ml/kg), relatively much higher than that for the cow, 50 ml/cow (0.1 ml/kg).

Figure 11.4: Example of the use of allometric dose and interval scaling worksheet using oxytetracycline 100 mg/ml.

Antibiotic	Toxic dose	Toxic effects
Ampicillin	25 mg/kg i.m. for 2 days	Fatal enteritis
	5 mg/kg i.m. for 2 days	Weight loss
	40 mg/kg s.c. for 4 days	40% fatal enteritis over next 2 weeks
	10 mg/kg orally for 6 days	50% fatal enteritis over next month
	8 mg/kg bid s.c.	Enteritis; previously also had penicillin
	>5 mg/kg orally via antibiotic-treated water for 3 days	Fatal enteritis in 7/11 rabbits
Penicillin	LD$_{50}$ 5.25 g/kg orally	Both acute and chronic toxicity (enteritis)
Cephalexin	200 mg/rabbit for 7 days	Diarrhoea
Lincomycin	100 mg orally (single dose) in 1.5–2.0 kg rabbits	66% mortality with enteritis
	24 mg/kg orally via antibiotic-treated water	90% mortality with enteritis
	30 mg/day orally in 2.0–2.5 kg rabbits	100% mortality with enteritis by 3 days
	1.3 mg/adult rabbit in feed for 3 days	30/130 rabbits died with enteritis
	0.2 mg/kg i.m. for 2 days	33% mortality in 2 days
Clindamycin	15 mg/kg orally for 3 days	100% mortality with enteritis
	5 mg/kg orally for 2 days	50% mortality with enteritis within 72 hours
	Single dose of 30 mg/kg i.v.	4/6 rabbits had fatal enteritis 12–14 days after treatment
Tylosin	100 mg/rabbit for 7 days	Diarrhoea
Erythromycin	3 g/l in drinking water for 7 days	Diarrhoea
Spectinomycin	1 g/l in drinking water for 7 days	Diarrhoea
Vancomycin	75 mg/kg i.v.	Acute toxicity with 100% mortality
Minocycline	30mg/kg i.m. for 3 days	Reduction in growth rate
Spiramycin	Acute oral LD$_{50}$ 4.85 g/kg	Nervous signs

Figure 11.5: Adverse effects of antibiotic treatment in rabbits. Adapted from Morris (1995) with permission.

There do not appear to be any detailed reports in the literature on adverse effects of amoxycillin, but manufacturers of amoxycillin do hear anecdotal reports of its use without apparent complications in rabbits (C Hoare, personal communication). Caution with amoxycillin is warranted, as shown by a single case investigated by the author. A 4 kg rabbit was given 75 mg of an injectable long-acting amoxycillin preparation. Two days later, the animal was found with circulatory collapse and diarrhoea; at necropsy the caecum was enlarged, contained fluid faeces and its mucosa was haemorrhagic. In the caecum, histological lesions were similar to those with clindamycin-induced enteritis, and *Clostridia difficile* enterotoxin was present.

As enterocolitis is such a problem, it should be noted that it has been prevented by oral administration of antibiotics that are not absorbed across the intestinal tract. Fatal enteritis in the rabbit normally caused by ampicillin at 20 mg/kg for 3 days was avoided by concurrent administration of gentamicin (10 mg/kg/day); and enteritis caused by lincomycin (30 mg/day orally for 3 days in 2.0–2.5 kg rabbits) was prevented by gentamicin (30 mg/day orally).

Another approach is to use ion-exchange resins, such as cholestyramine, to bind the clostridial toxins, and this has been shown to have a beneficial effect in clindamycin-induced enterotoxaemia in rabbits (Lipman *et al.*, 1992).

Fluoroquinolones
The fluoroquinolones are useful agents and the relative lack of incidence of induced enterocolitis at clinical dose rates is particularly noteworthy. In rabbits, 25 mg/kg enrofloxacin was given for 12 days as part of a reproductive toxicity assessment, without adverse effects. Pharmacokinetic studies on enrofloxacin in rabbits have shown 5 mg/kg twice a day orally gives effective tissue levels. The empirical drinking water concentration for dosing is 100 mg/l. However, as in other species, administration of fluoroquinolones to growing rabbits can cause cartilage defects, leading to lameness (Sharpnack *et al.*, 1994).

Tetracyclines
Relative to many other antibiotics, tetracyclines are often considered by clinicians to be useful and rela-

tively safe broad-spectrum antibiotics for use in rabbits, and many authors quote dose rates for oral administration of tetracyclines. Recent reports, however, have shown that the oral route is of little use. Administration of tetracycline in the drinking water of rabbits at concentrations up to 1600 mg/l produced low to undetectable serum levels, and water intake was reduced at the highest drug concentration.

The use of long-acting preparations of oxytetracycline in the rabbit has been recommended; however, different formulations of long-acting oxytetracycline differ markedly in the degree of tissue irritation they produce. Those preparations that are most irritant can cause visible distress to the animal, tissue damage, prolonged tissue residues, and the lowest and most delayed peak concentrations. This should be considered, as some pharmaceutical companies actively promote their formulations of long-acting oxytetracycline on the basis of lower tissue irritancy.

Sulphonamides
Caution is necessary with different trimethoprim-potentiated sulphonamide brands which may contain different sulphonamides, such as sulphadiazine. In the rabbit the half-life of this sulphonamide is only about an hour, compared to 5–10 hours in other species. In each country, different trimethoprim-potentiated sulphonamide brands are available, so it would be advisable for clinicians to confirm the sulphonamide in their usual brand.

Ocular antibiotics
Guidance on antibiotic selection for ocular infections is aided by a recent study where staphylococci were recently found as the commonest bacterial species isolated from rabbits with clinical signs of ocular infection (Cobb *et al., 1999*). A fusidic acid preparation has recently been approved in the UK for use for ocular staphylococcal infections in the rabbit (Fucithalmic Vet, Leo Animal Health). In general, aqueous presentations persist longer in the tear fluid of rabbits compared to dogs (van Busterveld *et al.*,1987). Based on minimal inhibitory concentrations (MICs) related to staphylococcal species, for 17 out of 18 isolates from rabbits' eyes, the MIC was found to be <4 g/ml (M Cobb, personal communication). The sustained release preparation of fusidic acid (Fucithalmic Vet, Leo Animal Health) would thus allow administration once or twice a day in order to have a >4 g/ml concentration in tear fluid at 24 hours (van Busterveld *et al.*, 1987). There is a potential for systemic absorption of antibiotics from topical presentations; however, ocular administration of fusidic acid to rabbits for 42 days does not cause local toxicity, nor were there signs of gastrointestinal side effects in rabbits given 125 mg fusidic acid a day from day 6 to day 18 of gestation, when it was used as part of a safety assessment for teratogenicity (M Cobb, personal communication).

Antiparasitic agents

Ivermectin
Ivermectin has been used extensively in rabbits for both ecto- and endoparasites (Soll, 1989). It is well distributed throughout the body after subcutaneous administration at 400 µg/kg, and persists for at least 2 weeks in significant concentrations (McKellar *et al.,* 1992). The large number of clinical reports, this background pharmacokinetic data, and the relative absence of published or anecdotal reports of toxicity, suggest ivermectin is safe and efficacious for parasite control in the rabbit.

Topical agents
More recently available topically applied agents, such as fipronil, while possibly efficacious, may not be suitably formulated for the rabbit. For example, one formulation of fipronil spray (Frontline Spray, Merial) is unsuitable for rabbits, probably because of the alcohol excipient (Cooper and Penaliggon, 1997).

Benzimidazoles
Benzimidazole anthelmintics have been widely used in the rabbit, especially thiabendazole and fenbendazole. Doses are available from formularies, may be on file at the drug's manufacturer and have been reviewed by Hofing and Kraus (1994), although they note, as with most rabbit therapies 'dosage information and efficacy information are not readily available'.

Anticoccidial drugs
Drugs to control coccidian parasites – sulphaquinoxaline, lasalocid and salinomycin – are licensed in some countries (Hayhow, 1998).

Vaccines
Several vaccines for myxomatosis and viral haemorrhagic disease virus-induced disease are available. Efficacy of myxomatosis vaccine can be reduced if the relatively unfamiliar intradermal route is not used for part of the dose. Attempts continue to produce a reliable vaccine against *Pasteurella multocida*, but currently none is available.

Drugs acting on the respiratory system
Due to the anatomical and pathological features of the nasolacrimal duct (see above), drugs instilled into the palpebral opening may overflow on to the skin adjacent to the lateral canthus of the eye, and may fail to get to the whole nasolacrimal tract. This may be of importance in *Pasteurella* sp. infections of the lacrimal sac.

Drugs acting on the gastrointestinal system
The enzyme bromelain, contained in pineapple juice, has been recommended for treatment of gastric trichobezoars. Current opinion tends toward the view that some hair in the stomach is not abnormal but that

larger trichobezoars are secondary to gastrointestinal motility disorders (see Chapter 5). As such, more rational treatment is fluid therapy and administration of liquefied fibre-rich diets and drugs that enhance intestinal motility. Metoclopramide is becoming widely used for this purpose, although drugs that have a greater effect on the large bowel, such as cisapride, may be more effective. No controlled studies of these approaches have been reported.

Drugs acting on the reproductive system

Rabbits do not have a regular oestrous cycle and are induced ovulators. Gonadotropin releasing hormone (GnRH) analogues, such as buserelin, are licensed for induction of ovulation for rabbit breeding enterprises in some countries (Hayhow, 1998), and their effective use has been well characterized (Bechstedt, 1989). Use of GnRH analogues avoids the problems that can be seen with repeated use of luteinizing hormone (LH), where anti-LH antibodies can be produced.

Drugs acting on the central nervous system

Some rabbits have high levels of atropine esterase, so glycopyrrolate has been suggested as an alternative to atropine (Olson *et al.*, 1993). Anaesthetics and analgesics are covered in Chapter 12.

REFERENCES

Anderson JA and Henk JW (1994) Toxicity and safety testing. In: *The Biology of the Laboratory Rabbit, 2nd edn*, ed. PJ Manning *et al.*, p.460. Academic Press, San Diego

Bechstedt U (1989) Use of Gonavet 'Berlin-Chemie' for ovulation in the rabbit with due consideration of different external heat symptoms. *Archiv für Tierzucht* **32**, 107-114

Brewer N R and Cruise LJ (1994) Physiology. In: *The Biology of the Laboratory Rabbit, 2nd edn*, ed. PJ Manning *et al.*, pp.66-67. Academic Press, San Diego

Cobb MA, Payne B, Allen WM and Pott JM (1999) A survey of the conjunctival flora in rabbits with clinical signs of superficial ocular infection. In: *Proceedings of the British Small Animal Veterinary Association Congress*, p.250. BSAVA, Cheltenham

Cooper PE and Penaliggon J (1997) Use of Frontline spray on rabbits. *Veterinary Record* **40**, 535-536

Cruise LJ and Brewer NR (1994) Anatomy. In: *The Biology of the Laboratory Rabbit, 2nd edn*, ed. PJ Manning *et al.*, pp. 54-56. Academic Press, San Diego

Davies B and Morris T (1993) Physiological parameters in laboratory animals and humans. *Pharmaceutical Research* **10**, 1093-1095

European Commission (1990) Council Directive 90/679, amending Directive 81/851/EEC on the approximation of the laws of the Member States relating to veterinary medicinal products. *Official Journal of the European Communities* L 373, (31/12/ 1990), 15-25

Evans RJ (1985) Clinical pharmacology and therapeutics. In: *Feline Medicine and Therapeutics, 2nd edn*, ed. EA Chandler *et al.*, pp.623-655. Blackwell Scientific, Oxford

Federal Register (1996) Animal Drug Availability Act 1996, Extralabel Drug Use in Animals; Final Rule. *Federal Register* **61**, (217), 57731-57746

Flecknell PA (1998) In: *The Veterinary Formulary, 4th edn*, ed Y Bishop, pp48-51 Pharmaceutical Press, London

Hawk CT and Leary S.K. (1999) *Formulary for Laboratory Animals, 2nd edn*. Iowa State University Press, Ames, Iowa

Hayhow C (1998) Drug availability for minor species in the 21st century: rabbits. *Veterinary and Human Toxicology* **40**, (suppl. 1), 28-29

Hillyer EV and Quesenberry KE (1997) *Ferrets, Rabbits and Rodents; Clinical Medicine and Surgery*. WB Saunders, Philadelphia

Hofing GL and Kraus AL (1994) Arthropod and helminth parasites. In: *The Biology of the Laboratory Rabbit, 2nd edn*, ed. PJ Manning *et al.*, p.243 Academic Press, San Diego

Johnson ET and Griffin KJ (1985) Variations in hepatic progesterone 21-hydroxylase activity reflect differences in the microsomal concentration of rabbit cytochrome P-450. *Archives of Biochemistry and Biophysics* **237**, 55-64

Johnson-Delaney CA (1996) In: *Exotic companion medicine handbook for veterinarians*, pp34-49. Wingers Publishing, Florida

Kararli TT (1995) Comparison of the gastrointestinal anatomy, physiology and biochemistry of humans and commonly used laboratory animals. *Biopharmaceutics and Drug Disposition* **16**, 351-380

Laber Laird K, Swindle MM and Flecknell P (1996) *Handbook of Rodent and Rabbit Medicine*. Pergamon, Oxford

Lave T, Portmann R, Schenker G, *et al.* (1999) Interspecies pharmacokinetic comparisons and allometric scaling of Napsagatran, a low molecular weight thrombin inhibitor. *Journal of Pharmacy & Pharmacology* **51**, 85-91

Lin JH (1998) Applications and limitations of interspecies scaling and in vitro extrapolation in pharmacokinetics. *Drug Metabolism and Disposition* **26**, 1202-1212

Lipman NS, Weischedel AK, Connors MJ, *et al.* (1992) Utilisation of cholestyramine resin as a preventative treatment for antibiotic (clindamycin) induced enterotoxaemia in the rabbit. *Laboratory Animals* **26**, 1-8

Marini RP, Foltz CJ, Kersten D, *et al.* (1996) Microbiologic, radiographic and anatomic study of the nasolacrimal duct apparatus in the rabbit (*Oryctolagus cuniculus*). *Laboratory Animal Science* **46**, 656-662

Martinez MN (1998a) Non compartmental methods of drug characterization: statistical moment theory. *Journal of the American Veterinary Medical Association* **213**, 974-980

Martinez MN (1998b) Volume, clearance and half-life. *Journal of the American Veterinary Medical Association* **213**, 1122-1127

Martinez MN (1998c) Physicochemical properties of pharmaceuticals. *Journal of the American Veterinary Medical Association* **213**, 1274-1277

Martinez MN (1998d) Clinical applications of pharmacokinetics. *Journal of the American Veterinary Medical Association* **213**, 1418-1420

Martinez MN (1998e) Clinically important errors in data interpretation. *Journal of the American Veterinary Medical Association* **213**, 1564-1569

McKeller QA, Midgley DM, Galbraith EA, *et al.* (1992) Clinical and pharmacological properties of ivermectin in rabbits and guinea pigs. *Veterinary Record* **130**, 71-73

Melich D (1990) A method for chronic intravenous infusion of the rabbit via the marginal ear vein. *Laboratory Animal Science* **40**, 327-328

Morris TH (1995) Antibiotic therapeutics in laboratory animals. *Laboratory Animals* **29**, 16-36

Morris TH (1999) Dose estimation among species. In: *Formulary for Laboratory Animals, 2nd edn*, ed. CT Hawk and SK Leary, pp. 3-14. Iowa State University Press, Ames, Iowa

Morris TH (2000) Anaesthesia in the fourth dimension. Is biological scaling relevant to veterinary anaesthesia? *Veterinary Anaesthesia and Analgesia* **27**, 2-5

Olson ME, Vizzutti D, Morck DW, *et al.* (1993) The parasympatholytic effects of atropine sulfate and glycopyrrolate in rats and rabbits. *Canadian Journal of Veterinary Research* **57**, 254-258

Ritschel WA and Hammer GV (1980) Prediction of the volume of distribution from in vitro data and use for estimating the absolute extent of absorption. *International Journal of Clinical Pharmacology, Therapy and Toxicology* **18**, 298-316

Riviere JE (1995) An AAVPT perspective: Part II. A review of the first interactive workshop on professional flexible labelling. *Journal of the American Veterinary Medical Association* **207**, 876-878

Riviere JE, Martin-Jimenez T, Syndfot SF, *et al.* (1997) Interspecies allometric analysis of the comparative pharmacokinetics of 44 drugs across veterinary and laboratory animal species. *Journal of Veterinary Pharmacology and Therapeutics.* **20**, 453-463

Rozman K (1988) Disposition of xenobiotics, species differences. *Toxicologic Pathology* **16**, 123-129

Sharpnack DD, Mastin JP, Childress CP, *et al.* (1994) Quinolone arthropathy in juvenile New Zealand White rabbits. *Laboratory Animal Science* **44**, 436-442

Smith RL (1974) The problem of species variation. *Annales de la Nutrition et de l'Alimentation* **28**, 335-349

Soll MD (1989) Use of ivermectin in laboratory and exotic mammals and in birds, fish and reptiles. In: *Ivermectin and Abamectin*, ed. WC Campbell, pp. 260-286. Springer-Verlag, New York

Tennant B (1999) (ed.) *BSAVA Small Animal Formulary, 3rd edn*. BSAVA, Cheltenham

van Busterveld OP, Andriesse H and Nielsen BH (1987) Fusidic acid in tear fluid: pharmacokinetic study with fusidic acid viscous eye drops. *European Journal of Drug Metabolism and Pharmacokinetics* **12,** 215–218

VMD (1995) *The Medicine (Restrictions on the Administration of Veterinary Medicinal Products) Regulations 1994 (SI 1994/2987), Guidance to the Veterinary Profession.* Amelia 8 Veterinary Medicines Directorate, Addlestone

Walker C (1978) Species differences in microsomal monoxgeneic activity and their relationship to biological half-lives. *Drug Metabolism Reviews* **7,** 295–323

West GB, Brown JH and Enquist BJ (1999) The fourth dimension of life: fractal geometry and the allometric scaling of organisms. *Science* **284,**1677–1679

Wolf CR, Smith BR, Ball LM, *et al.* (1979) The rabbit pulmonary monoxygenase system. *Journal of Biological Chemistry* **254,** 3658–3663

Wyss PA, Mühlebach S and Bickel MH (1982) Pharmacokinectics of 2,2′,4,4′,5,5′-Hexachlorobiphenyl (6-CB) in rats with decreasing adipose tissue mass. I. Effects of restricting food intake two weeks after administration of 6-CB. *Drug Metabolism and Disposition* **10,** 657–661

CHAPTER TWELVE

Anaesthesia

Paul A. Flecknell

INTRODUCTION

Successful anaesthesia of rabbits, as with any other species, requires careful attention to all aspects of perioperative care. There are a few specific issues that are of particular importance, for example the relative difficulty of endotracheal intubation and the apparent increased susceptibility to respiratory arrest, and these are discussed in the relevant sections below. Rabbits should not, however, be at special risk of anaesthetic-related complications once familiarity with the responses of this species to the anaesthetic agents and techniques used has been gained.

ANAESTHETIC EQUIPMENT

Since adult rabbits range in size from 500 g to over 10 kg, apparatus used in cats and small dogs is appropriate in most circumstances. Very small rabbits, such as juveniles or dwarf breeds, will benefit from the use of more specialized apparatus. Anaesthetic circuits should have a low dead space, and either a T-piece or Bain circuit is recommended. The tidal volume of anaesthetized rabbits is often only 5–10 ml/kg during spontaneous respiration, so low dead-space connectors, such as those used in human paediatric anaesthesia, are recommended for smaller rabbits (<2 kg) (Figure 12.1).

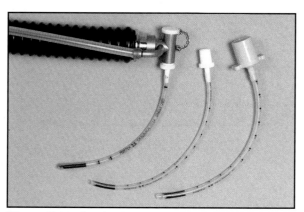

Figure 12.1: *A low dead-space endotracheal tube connector for use in smaller rabbits (<2 kg) and connector attached to paediatric T-piece. A standard connector is shown for comparison.*

High-risk patients, such as those with obvious respiratory infections or other clinical problems, may benefit from assisted ventilation. If the animal has been intubated (see below) this can be achieved manually, using an open-ended reservoir bag on the end of a Bain circuit or T-piece, or a mechanical ventilator can be used. Several ventilators capable of delivering low tidal volumes are now widely available.

If intubation is to be carried out under direct visualization of the larynx, then an otoscope with an appropriate-sized speculum (Figure 12.2) should be available. If a laryngoscope is to be used, then a Wisconsin blade, size 0, 1 or 2, will be required, depending upon the size of the rabbit. Uncuffed endotracheal tubes ranging from 2.5 to 5 mm (or larger) are needed, and < 2.5 mm for animals weighing under 600 g. These latter tubes need to be purchased from specialist manufacturers or made from catheters or other tubing.

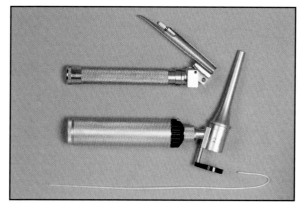

Figure 12.2: *Otoscope and laryngoscope (Wisconsin size 1 blade) for endotracheal intubation in the rabbit. Speculum sizes are suitable for a rabbit of 2–5 kg. The introducer for the endotracheal tube is shown at the bottom.*

PREANAESTHETIC PREPARATION

Clinical examination
A thorough clinical examination should be carried out, even with apparently healthy young animals undergoing elective surgery. Cardiac disease is rare, but respiratory infections are common. Respiratory rate is almost

invariably elevated during examination, often exceeding 200 breaths per minute, and it is preferable to observe the animal while it is resting, undisturbed, for any signs of dyspnoea. If abnormalities are detected, radiography may be required.

Fluid and electrolyte imbalances will frequently be present, e.g. in animals requiring anaesthesia for correction of dental disorders. Whenever possible these imbalances should be corrected before induction of anaesthesia. Since most anaesthetics reduce cardiac output and cause peripheral vasodilation, induction of anaesthesia in a dehydrated animal can rapidly lead to circulatory failure. Placement of intravenous catheters is usually achieved easily via the marginal ear veins (see Chapter 14) but use can also be made of the cephalic or mammary vessels (see Chapter 1). Generally, 'over-the-needle' style catheters are more reliable than 'butterfly' style infusion sets, as they are much less likely to become displaced through the vessel wall. Even in small rabbits (500 g), 23-24 gauge catheters can usually be placed in the ear veins.

Food and water

It is not necessary to withhold food or water for prolonged periods prior to anaesthesia. Indeed, it is preferable to encourage the animal to eat as this may minimize the risk of postoperative inappetence. Food should be removed about an hour before induction of anaesthesia, so that the mouth and pharynx will be free from food material.

Sedation and analgesia

Rabbits are easily stressed when placed in unfamiliar surroundings, and the restraint needed for induction of anaesthesia will also be stressful. This can increase the risk of complications during induction, alter the response to anaesthetic agents, and is distressing to the animal. For these reasons, some form of pre-anaesthetic medication is advisable and this should be integrated into the overall anaesthetic protocol. Agents such as acepromazine maleate, diazepam, midazolam, xylazine and medetomidine all produce sedation in the rabbit, and all of these agents markedly potentiate the effects of other anaesthetic agents. The dose rates, possible contraindications and effects of these agents are listed in Figure 12.3.

If surgery is to be undertaken, it may be advisable to incorporate an opioid analgesic in the preanaesthetic medication, especially if one is not to be used as part of the main anaesthetic protocol. Preanaesthetic administration of opioids may reduce the degree of pain experienced in the postoperative period, as well as reducing the dose of other anaesthetic agents needed. If non-steroidal anti-inflammatory drugs (NSAIDs) are to be used to provide analgesia (see below) then these should also be administered preoperatively, provided that blood pressure can be maintained to ensure adequate renal perfusion (Flecknell and Waterman-Pearson, in press). In other species, use of carprofen preoperatively has much less risk of causing such problems and it is reasonable to presume that similar benefits are seen in rabbits.

Drug	Dose rate	Comments
Acepromazine	0.1-0.5 mg/kg i.m.	Moderate to mild sedation Causes peripheral vasodilation Use with care in dehydrated animals, or those with cardiovascular disturbances
Atropine	50 micrograms/kg s.c. or i.m.	Ineffective in a high proportion of rabbits
Butorphanol/ acepromazine	1mg/kg + 0.5 mg/kg i.m.	Moderate sedation Causes peripheral vasodilation and some analgesia Use with care in dehydrated animals, or those with cardiovascular disturbances
Diazepam	1-2 mg/kg i.m. or i.p.	Moderate to deep sedation Use emulsion formulation to minimize risk of thrombophlebitis if administering i.v.
Glycopyrrolate	0.01 mg/kg i.v. 0.1 mg/kg s.c. or i.m.	Administer to reduce salivation and bronchial secretions and to prevent vagally mediated bradycardia
Fentanyl/fluanisone (Hypnorm)	0.2-0.5 ml/kg i.m.	Mild to profound sedation and moderate to marked analgesia (sufficient for minor surgery) Respiratory depression can be marked at high dose rates
Fentanyl/droperidol (Innovar Vet)	0.22 ml/kg i.m.	Mild to profound sedation and moderate to marked analgesia (sufficient for minor surgery) Respiratory depression can be marked at high dose rates
Ketamine	25-50 mg/kg i.m.	Moderate to heavy sedation Some analgesia

Figure 12.3: Suggested dose rates of preanaesthetic agents for use in the rabbit.   ▶

Drug	Dose rate	Comments
Ketamine	25–50 mg/kg i.m.	Moderate to heavy sedation Some analgesia
Medetomidine	0.1–0.5 mg/kg i.m. or s.c.	Mild to profound sedation Peripheral vasoconstriction can make subsequent venepuncture difficult Can cause respiratory and cardiovascular depression, so best avoided in animals in poor health
Midazolam	2 mg/kg i.v., i.m. or i.p.	Moderate to deep sedation Water-soluble
Xylazine	5 mg/kg i.m.	Mild to profound sedation Peripheral vasoconstriction can make subsequent venepuncture difficult Can cause respiratory and cardiovascular depression, so best avoided in animals in poor health

Figure 12.3 continued: Suggested dose rates of preanaesthetic agents for use in the rabbit.

Often, sedation and analgesia can be provided by administering one component of a balanced anaesthetic regimen to the rabbit while it is still in its cage, followed by use of additional agents after transfer to the operating theatre. Examples are fentanyl/fluanisone followed 10 minutes later by diazepam or midazolam, and medetomidine followed 5 minutes later by ketamine. The reason for not administering all of the components of the anaesthetic regimen together, is that it is strongly advisable to administer oxygen during induction of anaesthesia, and this is most easily achieved after the sedated rabbit has been transferred to theatre.

Anticholinergic agents

It is not usually necessary to administer anticholinergic agents to reduce salivary and bronchial secretions, or to reduce bradycardia due to vagal reflexes. However, if bradycardia occurs during abdominal or cervical surgery, then it can be corrected or prevented by the use of glycopyrrolate (0.01–0.1 mg/kg). Atropine is ineffective in a large proportion of rabbits (up to 50% of some strains) because of the production of atropinesterase which rapidly degrades atropine. High doses of atropine (1–2 mg/kg) may be effective, but additional doses may be needed every 10–15 minutes. Since the atropinesterase levels in a particular individual will be uncertain, it is best to avoid giving such large doses of atropine, and either use glycopyrrolate, or administer a small dose of atropine (0.05 mg/kg) and assess the effect, and give additional doses if required.

INDUCTION AND MAINTENANCE OF ANAESTHESIA

Typically, a discussion of the selection of anaesthetic regimens is structured in terms of route of administration or broad class of agent. This structure reinforces the misconception that use of single anaesthetic agents,

at high doses, is the preferred means of anaesthetizing an animal. This is not correct in any species, but in the rabbit adoption of this approach has probably contributed to the high mortality reported in this species (Clark and Hall, 1999). Two commonly used induction agents, alphaxalone/alphadolone (Saffan, Schering-Plough Animal Health) and propofol, when used alone, only produce surgical anaesthesia at dose rates that are close to those that cause respiratory arrest. Induction and maintenance with a volatile agent may also be hazardous, since all of the commonly available inhalational anaesthetics provoke breath-holding and bradycardia in rabbits (Flecknell et al., 1996). Balanced anaesthesia, in which a combination of agents are administered, usually at relatively low doses, is therefore particularly appropriate for use in the rabbit.

When selecting an anaesthetic regimen, it is advisable to develop expertise with one or two techniques, and adapt these for particular purposes or for higher risk patients. The following techniques are suggested for routine use. A more comprehensive listing of agents, dose rates and effects are given in Figure 12.4. With all of the injectable anaesthetic regimens, oxygen must be administered either by face mask, via an endotracheal tube, or by use of a nasal catheter or placement of a catheter in the pharynx via the mouth.

Anaesthetic regimens

Option 1: Medetomidine plus ketamine

Medetomidine (0.25 mg/kg s.c.) is given to sedate the animal. Five minutes later, oxygen can be given by mask to the animal, followed by ketamine (15 mg/kg s.c. or i.m.). Alternatively, the two drugs can be mixed and administered as a single injection.

Rabbits lose consciousness within 10–15 minutes of receiving both drugs. Endotracheal intubation can then be carried out, as laryngeal relaxation is usually good. This regimen produces moderate peripheral

Anaesthetic	Dose rate	Comments
Alphaxalone/alphadolone	6–9 mg/kg i.v.	Light anaesthesia, 5–10 min Apnoea common at higher dose rates Sleep time 10–20 min
Fentanyl/fluanisone + diazepam	0.3 ml/kg i.m. + 2 mg/kg i.p. or i.v.	Surgical anaesthesia, 20–40 min Good relaxation Sleep time 60–120 min Some of effects reversible (see text)
Fentanyl/fluanisone + midazolam	0.3 ml/kg i.m. + 2 mg/kg i.m. or i.v.	Surgical anaesthesia, 20–40 min Good relaxation Sleep time 60–120 min Some of effects reversible (see text)
Ketamine/acepromazine	50 mg/kg i.m. + 1 mg/kg i.m.	Surgical anaesthesia, 20–30 min Good relaxation Sleep time 60–120 min
Ketamine/diazepam	25 mg/kg i.m. + 5 mg/kg i.m.	Surgical anaesthesia, 20–30 min Good relaxation Sleep time 60–120 min
Ketamine/medetomidine	15 mg/kg s.c. + 0.25 mg/kg s.c.	Surgical anaesthesia, 20–30 min Good relaxation Sleep time 90–180 min Some of effects reversible (see text)
Ketamine/medetomidine/ butorphanol	15 mg/kg s.c. + 0.25 mg/kg s.c. + 0.4 mg/kg s.c.	Surgical anaesthesia, 30–40 min Good relaxation Sleep time 90–240 min Some of effects reversible (see text)
Ketamine/xylazine	35 mg/kg i.m. + 5 mg/kg i.m.	Surgical anaesthesia, 20–30 min Good relaxation Sleep time 60–120 min Some of effects reversible (see text)
Ketamine/xylazine/ butorphanol	50 mg/kg i.m. + 5 mg/kg i.m. + 0.1 mg/kg i.m.	Surgical anaesthesia, 60–90 min Good relaxation Sleep time 120–180 min
Ketamine/xylazine/ acepromazine	35 mg/kg i.m. + 5 mg/kg i.m. + 1 mg/kg i.m.	Surgical anaesthesia, 45–75 min Good relaxation Sleep time 100–150 min
Pentobarbitone	30–45 mg/kg i.v. (not recommended)	Light to medium planes of anaesthesia, 20–30 min Higher doses have high risk of respiratory and cardiac arrest Sleep time 60–120 min
Propofol	10 mg/kg i.v.	Light anaesthesia, 5–10 min Apnoea common at higher dose rates Recovery smooth and rapid Sleep time 10–15 min
Thiopentone	30 mg/kg i.v.	Surgical anaesthesia, 5–10 min Sleep time 10–15 min

Figure 12.4: *Anaesthetic and analgesic doses for rabbits. Note that most drugs do not have a product licence and that individual variations in responses may occur. All injectable anaesthetics cause respiratory depression in rabbits, and oxygen should be administered to prevent hypoxia. Great care should be exercised when using fixed-dose combinations in animals with possible compromised cardiovascular or respiratory function, or other disorders.*

vasoconstriction, so peripheral venepuncture or placement of an over-the-needle catheter is less straightforward than when other regimens are used. The peripheral vasoconstriction also produces a pale and bluish coloration of the mucous membranes, even when oxygen is administered to prevent hypoxia. If oxygen is not provided, then marked cyanosis is often apparent (Figure 12.5). In other species, this combination produces moderate cardiovascular depression, so it is not advisable for use as a routine regimen in animals with pre-existing fluid deficits. It is a very useful means of anaesthetizing rabbits which are in overt good health, as the main complication, hypoxia, can be corrected easily by administration of oxygen. Only moderate hypercapnia develops after anaesthesia with this regimen and this is easily corrected by intubation and assisted ventilation if anaesthesia is to be prolonged.

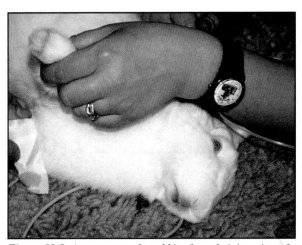

Figure 12.5: Appearance of a rabbit after administration of medetomidine (0.25 mg/kg s.c.) combined with ketamine (15 mg/kg s.c.). Oxygen should always be administered to prevent hypoxia.

In most animals, surgical anaesthesia is produced for 30–60 minutes. The duration of anaesthesia can be prolonged by the addition of butorphanol (0.1 mg/kg) or buprenorphine (0.05 mg/kg) to the ketamine/medetomidine regimen, resulting in approximately 80 minutes of surgical anaesthesia. If insufficient analgesia is produced, or an animal becomes too lightly anaesthetized during a prolonged procedure, it is possible to deepen anaesthesia by administration of additional ketamine and medetomidine, at approximately a third of the original dose, but this is not advisable. It is preferable to provide additional analgesia, either by using 0.5–1% of halothane or isoflurane, or by infiltrating the surgical site with local anaesthetic. If additional ketamine and medetomidine are to be used to prolong anaesthesia, then these should be administered at approximately one tenth of the original dose, diluted 1:10 with water for injection, by slow intravenous injection, until the desired effect is achieved.

This regimen has the particular advantage of being partially reversed when atipamezole is administered. Ketamine used alone at the dose rates stated in Figure 12.3 produces immobility and a mild degree of analgesia for approximately 45–60 minutes. Consequently, administration of atipamezole when ketamine/medetomidine has been used results in very rapid recovery (Figure 12.6). It is this feature that makes the combination so attractive, but since its administration frequently results in severe hypoxia, oxygen should always be administered to prevent this. It is worth noting that the agent's effects are clearly dose dependent, so the mixture can be used to provide light anaesthesia for procedures such as radiography (0.2 mg/kg medetomidine plus 10 mg/kg ketamine s.c.) or initial sedation and immobilization followed by use of low concentrations of inhalant agents to produce full surgical anaesthesia.

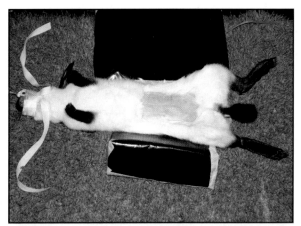

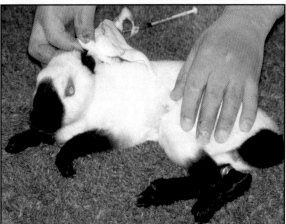

Figure 12.6: (a) A rabbit anaesthetized with ketamine (15 mg/kg s.c.) and medetomidine (0.25 mg/kg s.c.) for ovariohysterectomy. A heating pad has been placed beneath the bedding. (b) Appearance of the animal 5 minutes after administration of atipamezole. (NB Carprofen was administered preoperatively to provide postoperative analgesia).

Ketamine (35 mg/kg i.m.) combined with xylazine (5 mg/kg i.m.) can be used, but the degree of analgesia produced is slightly less than when medetomidine is administered.

Option 2: Fentanyl/fluanisone plus midazolam or diazepam

Fentanyl/fluanisone (Hypnorm, Janssen–Cilag) (0.3 ml/kg i.m.) is followed approximately 5–10 minutes later by midazolam (1–2 mg/kg) or diazepam (1–2 mg/kg) by intravenous or intramuscular injection.

Since the administration of Hypnorm produces vasodilation, as well as profound analgesia and sedation, venepuncture is made easier, even in very small rabbits. Intravenous injection enables the drugs to be given to effect so that a lower total dose of midazolam or diazepam is administered. This results in a more rapid recovery. If diazepam is to be administered intravenously, then it is preferable to use an emulsion preparation rather than formulations containing propylene glycol, as these are associated with a low risk of thrombophlebitis at the site of injection.

The combination of Hypnorm and midazolam or diazepam produces surgical anaesthesia and good muscle relaxation, lasting 30–45 minutes. Recovery can be prolonged (up to 3 hours) but can be shortened by administering butorphanol (0.1–0.5 mg/kg s.c. or i.v.), buprenorphine (0.01–0.05 mg/kg s.c. or i.v.), or another mixed agonist/antagonist opioid (Figure 12.7). Butorphanol is an antagonist at mu opioid receptors, so reverses the effects of fentanyl, but since it is also an agonist at kappa receptors, some continued analgesia is provided. Buprenorphine also reverses the effects of fentanyl, but its effects are less pronounced than those of butorphanol, although it provides a much longer period of postoperative analgesia (6–8 hours compared to 2–3 hours; Flecknell and Liles, 1990).

If a rabbit is insufficiently anaesthetized or anaesthesia lightens during surgery, additional Hypnorm can be administered by intramuscular injection (typically, approximately one third of the original dose). More accurate supplementation can be achieved by administering additional Hypnorm by intravenous injection, but the commercial preparation should first be diluted 1:10 with water for injection (saline can result in formation of small crystals in the diluted solution) so that it can be given slowly, in a controlled way.

Rabbits anaesthetized with Hypnorm plus diazepam or midazolam develop moderate hypoxia and hypercapnia, and should be given oxygen throughout the period of anaesthesia. It is important to note that the similar neuroleptanalgesic combination Innovar Vet (Mallinckrodt, USA) (fentanyl/droperidol) does *not* produce equivalent effects when combined with diazepam or midazolam, and this combination cannot be used to anaesthetize rabbits safely.

Option 3: Propofol or thiopentone followed by halothane or isoflurane

Induction with propofol (10 mg/kg i.v.) or thiopentone (30 mg/kg i.v. of 1.25% solution – note the hazard of extravascular administration, see below) may be followed by maintenance with halothane or isoflurane.

Other anaesthetic combinations

Ketamine (50 mg/kg) and acepromazine (1 mg/kg); and ketamine (25 mg/kg) and midazolam or diazepam (5 mg/kg): These combinations, administered by intramuscular injection, usually produce light to moderate surgical anaesthesia, for 20–30 minutes. Recovery times are normally 1–2 hours. These anaesthetic mixtures often fail to produce surgical anaesthesia, so are best used for relatively non-painful interventions, such as radiography. The degree of respiratory depression is less than with other combinations (that provide deeper planes of anaesthesia) but oxygen should still be administered. The addition of acepromazine to the ketamine/xylazine or ketamine/medetomidine combinations increases the duration of anaesthesia (see Figure 12.4). Tiletamine/zolezepam can be used to provide light to moderate anaesthesia in rabbits, but its use has been associated with the development of renal damage and so it should be avoided in this species (Lipman *et al.*, 1997).

Analgesic	Dose rate	Estimated duration of action
Opioids		
Buprenorphine	0.01–0.05 mg/kg s.c.or i.v.	6–12 hours
Butorphanol	0.1–0.5 mg/kg s.c. or i.v.	2–4 hours
Pethidine (Meperidine)	5–10 mg/kg i.m. or s.c.	2–4 hours
Nalbuphine	1–2 mg/kg i.v.	4 hours
NSAIDs		
Carprofen	1.5 mg/kg orally, 1–2 mg/kg s.c. or i.v.	?24 hours
Flunixin	1.1 mg/kg s.c.	?12–24 hours
Ketoprofen	3 mg/kg i.m.	?12–24 hours
Meloxicam	0.2–0.3 mg/kg orally, 0.2 mg/kg s.c.	?24 hours

Figure 12.7: Analgesics for use in the rabbit. Suggested dose rates are based on clinical experience of the author and other colleagues. None of these agents has a veterinary product licence for use in the rabbit. Effects will vary in individual animals, and each rabbit should be assessed to try to determine the efficacy of the analgesic.

Propofol (10 mg/kg i.v.): This is less effective in the rabbit than in other species, and only light anaesthesia is produced at this dose rate (Glen, 1980). Higher doses (15–20 mg/kg) cause respiratory arrest. Propofol is useful as an induction agent and provides sufficient depth of anaesthesia for intubation. As in other species, recovery is rapid and reasonably smooth and free from excitement. Attempts to produce prolonged anaesthesia in rabbits with propofol have been less successful than in other species (Blake *et al.*, 1988; Ko, *et al.*, 1992; Aeschbacher and Webb, 1993a,b).

Alphaxalone/alphadolone (6–9 mg/kg i.v.): This produces similar effects to propofol, i.e. light general anaesthesia with sufficient relaxation for intubation. Recovery is less smooth. At the higher dose rates necessary to produce medium or deep surgical anaesthesia, sudden apnoea can occur (Green *et al.*, 1978) and, in contrast to propofol, this may rapidly be followed by cardiac arrest. This anaesthetic is not recommended for the rabbit.

Thiopentone (30 mg/kg i.v., using a 1.25% solution) or methohexitone (10–15 mg/kg i.v., using a 1% solution): Both these can be used as induction agents, enabling endotracheal intubation and maintenance with volatile anaesthetics. If used alone they produce 5–10 minutes of light to moderate anaesthesia. Recovery is often associated with excitement unless a suitable preanaesthetic medication has been given (e.g. acepromazine). As in other species, extravascular administration of thiopentone can cause severe thrombophlebitis.

Pentobarbitone (30–45 mg/kg i.v.): If this must be used, it should be diluted to provide a 30 mg/ml solution and administered slowly to effect. Considerable skill and extensive practical experience is required to use this drug effectively in the rabbit. Respiratory arrest frequently occurs before the onset of surgical anaesthesia and because of the consequent high mortality associated with its use, this drug is best avoided in this species (Flecknell *et al.*, 1983; Peeters *et al.,* 1988).

EMLA cream: If intravenous induction is planned, or if an 'over-the-needle' catheter is to be placed to allow preoperative fluid therapy, EMLA cream (Astra Zeneca) can be used to facilitate venepuncture. EMLA is a mixture of lignocaine and prilocaine that produces full skin-thickness anaesthesia. The fur overlying the ear vein is plucked or shaved, and a 2–3 mm thick layer of EMLA applied (Figure 12.8). This is then covered with a plastic film dressing (Figure 12.9) and a bandage. The dressing is removed after approximately 45 minutes and venepuncture carried out. As the skin has been anaesthetized, the animal does not react when the needle punctures the vein.

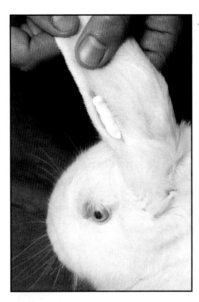

Figure 12.8: EMLA cream applied over the peripheral ear vein.

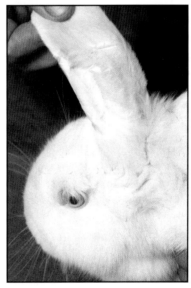

Figure 12.9: The EMLA cream is covered with a plastic dressing, then an outer bandage.

Use of volatile anaesthetics

Halothane or isoflurane

Halothane or isoflurane can be used to maintain effective and safe anaesthesia in the rabbit. Unfortunately, induction with these agents is often associated with prolonged breath-holding, which may go unnoticed because of the firm physical restraint used. If inhalational agents are to be used for induction, the rabbit should be observed closely and the face-mask removed if breath-holding occurs, then replaced when breathing recommences. Since struggling can cause injury to the vertebrae (see Chapter 1), it is preferable to administer a sedative or tranquillizer before induction. These agents do not prevent breath-holding, but usually prevent the animal from struggling. It has been suggested that doxapram should be administered prior to administration of volatile anaesthetics, as this will prevent breath-holding and so speed induction. It is important to note that the breath-holding and struggling are due to the rabbit's attempting to avoid inhalation of volatile anaesthetics, presumably because the experience is unpleasant and causes distress. Removing the animal's control of its respiration by administering doxapram does not seem an appropriate and humane means of dealing with this problem. However, if use of a volatile agent is thought to be the safest means of inducing anaesthesia in a particular patient, then this technique may be judged acceptable. In most circumstances, use of a sedative or tranquillizer to reduce the degree of stress is more appropriate.

Nitrous oxide

Nitrous oxide has relatively low potency in rabbits, so there is little advantage to using it as a component of a balanced anaesthetic regimen. At best, 60% nitrous oxide will reduce the concentration of volatile anaesthetic needed for maintenance by 0.25–0.5%, and has little apparent effect in potentiating the effects of injectable agents. In view of the high incidence of respiratory disease in rabbits, it is preferable to administer 100% oxygen, rather than a mixture containing nitrous oxide. In addition, nitrous oxide is not removed by the activated charcoal used in many gas-scavenging systems, so health and safety considerations may also influence its use.

Endotracheal intubation

One of the most common problems encountered during anaesthesia of rabbits is respiratory arrest. It is difficult to assist ventilation using a face-mask or by manual compression of the thorax. Placement of an endotracheal tube helps to maintain a patent airway, and enables ventilation to be assisted easily and effectively should this be necessary.

Intubation can be carried out using one of three techniques. Before attempting any of these, oxygen should be administered for 1–2 minutes. It is normally preferable to use an uncuffed endotracheal tube, as this allows a tube with a slightly larger internal diameter to be used. In larger rabbits (>5 kg), cuffed tubes (>4 mm internal diameter) can be used.

Laryngoscope

One option for intubation is to use a Wisconsin laryngoscope blade to visualize the larynx, so that an introducer and endotracheal tube can be placed in the trachea under direct vision. This technique is relatively simple but requires the purchase of specialized equipment (see Figure 12.2) since other designs of laryngoscope blade are not as suitable.

Otoscope

A more practicable alternative is to use an otoscope to visualize the larynx (Figure 12.10). A medium-sized speculum is suitable for rabbits of 2–4 kg, and smaller or larger sizes for other body weights. After placing the rabbit on its back, the otoscope is advanced through the

gap between the incisor and cheek teeth into the pharynx until the larynx can be seen. It is possible to advance the speculum into the oesophagus if the tip of the epiglottis is positioned on the nasal aspect of the soft palate. To avoid this, the soft palate can be pushed with the otoscope tip to disengage the epiglottis. As the speculum is advanced, the paler triangle of the epiglottis can often be seen through the end of the soft palate, alerting the anaesthetist to the need to manipulate the structure. In many cases the larynx is clearly visible immediately, and an introducer can be passed through the otoscope into the larynx and on into the trachea. If a purpose-made introducer is not available, then a bitch or cat urinary catheter can be used, depending upon the size of the rabbit. If a catheter is used, the Luer fitting should be removed before use since this will not pass through the tip of the otoscope. After placing the introducer, the otoscope is removed, taking care not to change the position of the introducer. The endotracheal tube (2.5–3 mm for 2–3 kg rabbits) is then threaded on to the end of the introducer and advanced into the trachea. The introducer is withdrawn and the tube tied in position.

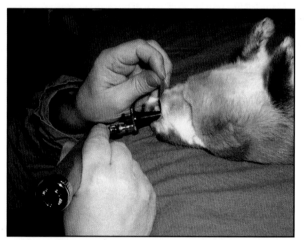

Figure. 12.10: *Use of an otoscope to view the larynx for endotracheal intubation.*

Blind technique

An alternative approach is to hold the rabbit as shown in Figure 12.11. The endotracheal tube is advanced through the gap between the incisors and premolars, and passed slowly down towards the larynx. Either the breath sounds can be monitored by listening at the end of the tube (Figure 12.11) or, if a clear polyethylene tube is used, condensation can be observed with each breath inside the tube. As the tube approaches the larynx, the sounds become louder, and if the tube passes down into the airway a small cough is often heard. If the tube passes into the oesophagus, then breath sounds (or condensation) are no longer apparent. In this case the tube should be withdrawn slightly, the head repositioned by tilting it either further back or slightly forwards, and the tube advanced again. In some instances, intubation can be made easier by use of local anaesthetic spray. This can be delivered on to the larynx by positioning the endotracheal tube at the point of maximal breath sounds, and then spraying lignocaine, or injecting a small (0.1 ml) quantity of lignocaine into the end of the tube. The local anaesthetic is drawn down the tube as the rabbit inhales and some reaches the larynx. After waiting a minute or two to allow the drug to act (preoxygenation can be repeated to this stage), another attempt at intubation can be made. If problems are encountered, oxygen should be administered every 4 minutes to ensure the animal does not become hypoxic.

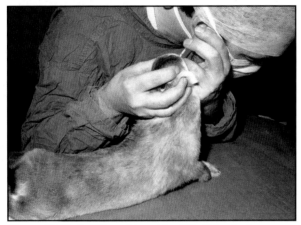

Figure 12.11: Rabbit positioned for 'blind' intubation.

Although this technique sounds challenging, it is relatively easy to become proficient, and the technique has the advantage of requiring no additional equipment. Although a modified stethoscope can be used to assist placement, with practice an operator can detect differences in resistance to tube passage that indicate successful placement. To confirm successful placement, condensation of breath on a cold surface, or movement of a few rabbit hairs placed at the end of the tube can be observed. In small rabbits (<1 kg) it is not always possible to hear breath sounds or observe condensation because of the small size of endotracheal tube (2–2.5 mm) that is needed. For this reason it is best to first gain proficiency by intubating larger rabbits. Whichever method of intubation is used, it is recommended that the rabbit be allowed to breathe 100% oxygen for 1–2 minutes before carrying out the procedure.

ANAESTHETIC MANAGEMENT AND INTRAOPERATIVE CARE

The general principles of good intraoperative care that apply to other species should be followed when anaesthetizing rabbits. Care should be taken to monitor adequate functioning of the circulatory and respiratory systems, and the animal's body temperature should be maintained. Most of the monitoring techniques used in the dog and cat can be used in larger rabbits but difficulties may be encountered in smaller animals (<2 kg).

Respiratory monitoring

The thermistor sensors which are used in most respiratory monitors are triggered reliably by rabbits weighing over 500 g but when respiration is depressed the instrument may fail to function. A better indication of respiratory function can be gained by using a pulse oximeter. These generally function well in most rabbits with the probe positioned across a toe in larger animals, or across the tail after shaving the fur (Figure 12.12) or on the tongue. Placement on the ear is generally less reliable, but it is advisable to try several positions, as different probe designs and different instruments seem to have sites at which they perform optimally. Although pulse oximeters generally function well, they are susceptible to signal loss caused by peripheral vasoconstriction, especially in smaller rabbits. This is a common problem when anaesthesia is produced using ketamine/ medetomidine or ketamine/xylazine.

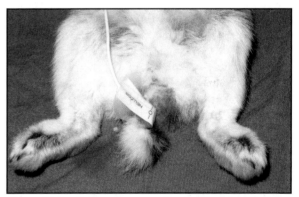

Figure 12.12: Pulse oximeter probe placed on the tail of a rabbit.

A second problem is that many instruments were originally designed for use in people and have an upper heart rate limit of 250 beats per minute. This is frequently exceeded in many rabbits. Some instruments will continue to register an accurate oxygen saturation level but others may simply display an error message at high heart rates. Heart rate in 2–4 kg rabbits is typically 200–280 beats per minute during anaesthesia with halothane, isoflurane or Hypnorm/midazolam (or diazepam). If medetomidine is used as preanaesthetic medication, or ketamine/medetomidine used for anaesthesia, heart rates will normally be 120–160 beats per minute. If possible it is helpful to assess an instrument before purchase, and in many instances instruments designed for veterinary use are to be preferred. Several of these have upper heart rate limits of 300–350 beats per minute or greater, and so can be used to their full potential with small mammals.

Respiratory depression

If respiratory depression occurs, as in larger species it can be treated by assisting ventilation and use of respiratory stimulants such as doxapram. It is advisable to administer oxygen immediately following induction of anaesthesia with injectable anaesthetics, since all of the agents used produce some degree of respiratory depression. In many instances severe hypoxia occurs and, if uncorrected, can lead to cardiac failure.

Provided the rabbit has been intubated, ventilation can be assisted easily in an emergency by intermittently occluding the outflow from a T-piece or Bain circuit, or preferably by gently squeezing the reservoir bag. If the rabbit has not been intubated, the animal should be positioned on its back with its head and neck in extension, oxygen delivered using a face-mask, and the chest compressed gently, approximately 40-60 times per minute. Attempts to ventilate the lungs using a face-mask are often relatively ineffective, and result in inflation of the stomach, rather than the lungs.

Cardiovascular monitoring

Pulse oximetry will provide some indication of cardio-vascular function. Cardiac function can also be monitored using a suitable ECG; an instrument capable of detecting low signal strengths and high frequencies is needed. Non-invasive blood pressure monitors are of little practicable value in rabbits but invasive blood pressure monitoring, via a catheter placed in the central ear artery, can be extremely valuable in high-risk patients (Figure 12.13). Clinical assessment of circulatory function can be made using capillary refill time, but palpation of peripheral pulses is not practicable except in larger rabbits.

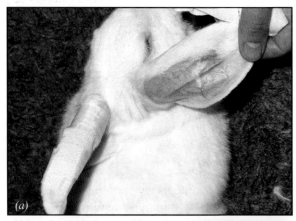

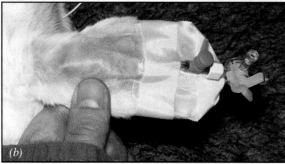

Figure 12.13: (a) The central ear artery. The overlying hair has been clipped and EMLA cream applied for 45 minutes before being wiped away. (b) A 22 gauge 'over-the-needle' catheter has been inserted, to allow measurement of arterial blood pressure.

Circulatory failure

Techniques for supporting the circulation or treating cardiac arrest are similar to those described for larger animals. Adrenaline can be used to treat low blood pressure and cardiac arrest associated with asystole. Arrhythmias can be treated with lignocaine or similar agents. As in other species, it is not advisable to treat the bradycardia which occurs following use of medetomidine with atropine because of the risk of causing severe hypertension. If bradycardia is so severe as to be considered life-threatening, atipamezole should be used and anaesthesia maintained using alternative anaesthetic agents.

Fluid or blood lost should be replaced; the general principles of therapy used in the dog and the cat can also be followed in rabbits.

Whole citrated blood from a donor rabbit can be used to restore blood volume after haemorrhage. Donor rabbits can provide 10-15% of their circulating volume (calculated as 65 ml/kg of body weight – so an adult 5 kg rabbit could provide 30-50 ml) for transfusion, and this can be collected in bags containing ACD (acid citrate dextrose) solution (1 part ACD to 3.5 parts whole blood) as for other species. There is little information concerning the frequency of adverse reactions to blood transfusion but in the author's experience initial transfusions from a single donor of the same breed do not seem associated with significant problems. If whole blood is unavailable, previously stored plasma or plasma substitutes can be administered. Other fluids (e.g. lactated Ringer's solution or Normal saline) can be used to correct fluid deficits as appropriate.

If fluid or blood loss is anticipated, for example during prolonged surgery, an infusion of warm (39 °C) lactated Ringer's solution should be established, at a rate of 10-15 ml/kg/h. After most surgical procedures, if fluids have not been administered intraoperatively, it is usually beneficial to administer warmed (39 °C) subcutaneous or intraperitoneal dextrose/saline at the end of surgery to provide some fluid supplementation in the immediate postoperative period.

In very small rabbits, or animals with severe vaso-constriction, fluid can be administered by the intraosseous route (see Chapter 1).

Maintenance of body temperature and general care

The rabbit's body temperature should be maintained (at 39 °C) throughout anaesthesia and during recovery. Even a small decrease in body temperature can significantly prolong recovery from anaesthesia and this is undesirable. Small rabbits (<1 kg) are particularly at risk of developing severe hypothermia and this can be life threatening if not corrected. To reduce the risk of hypothermia, clipping of the hair around the surgical site should be kept to a minimum compatible with aseptic technique.

Similarly, excessive use of skin disinfectants should be avoided. Body temperature can be conserved by use of 'bubble-wrap' or other insulating materials, and supplemental heat provided by heating blankets. It is bad practice to perform any surgery with the animal lying directly on the metal of an operating table.

Rabbits' eyes are prominent and the cornea can easily be abraded or become dry during anaesthesia. To avoid this, the eyelids may be taped closed using micropore tape, or an ophthalmic ointment may be applied (Figure 12.14). Ocular reflexes are of little assistance in assessing anaesthetic depth in rabbits, except to diagnose cardiac arrest and death! In many instances, palpebral responses are maintained even at deep planes of surgical anaesthesia. The most useful and reliable method of assessing depth of anaesthesia is by means of the hindlimb pedal withdrawal and ear pinch responses. Abolition of a response to an ear pinch and reduction of the pedal withdrawal response so that it is absent or barely detectable enables surgery to be carried out. Forelimb pedal withdrawal responses are lost at even deeper planes of anaesthesia, and it is not generally necessary or desirable to produce this degree of depression.

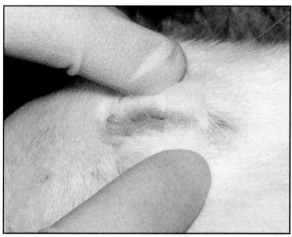

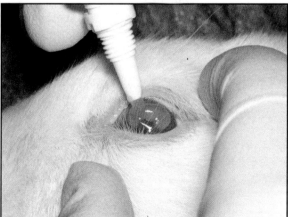

Figure 12.14: To prevent desiccation of the eyes during anaesthesia, the eyelids may be taped closed (a) or an ointment applied (b).

POSTOPERATIVE CARE

Provision of the most appropriate environmental conditions for recovery from surgery will improve the general comfort of the rabbit, reduce fear and anxiety, and increase the likelihood of the animal's making an uneventful recovery.

Environment

Fear and anxiety increase the degree of pain perceived by people and increase the requirement for analgesic therapy. It is likely that similar effects occur in animals, so measures to minimize fear and anxiety should be considered an essential part of nursing care. It is easy to overlook the effects on a rabbit of housing it in close proximity to a predator such as a cat or dog. In addition to preventing direct interaction between patients, remember that rabbits may also be affected by the odours remaining in the cage or recovery pen, or by odours on the clinician's hands or clothing. This can be prevented by effective cleaning of pens and by carrying out nursing procedures on 'prey' species before dealing with 'predators'.

Some rabbits respond positively to human contact, so nursing care, stroking, grooming and other forms of attention can be helpful. The response varies between individual animals, and it is important to select an appropriate level of care and attention.

It is essential that monitoring and support is provided in the postoperative period. Rabbits should be placed in a warm environment, that is draught free. Warm, comfortable bedding should be provided. Sawdust or wood shavings are *not* suitable. Once the animal has regained activity it can be transferred to a cage or pen containing plenty of good quality hay or straw. This type of bedding allows the animal to surround itself with insulating material, which provides both warmth and a sense of security, and also gives an immediate source of food.

Food and fluids

Animals should be encouraged to eat and drink as soon as possible after recovery from anaesthesia, unless there is a specific contraindication, but care must be taken that they do not spill water bowls – if the animal becomes wet it will lose heat rapidly. Since many rabbits have a reduced fluid intake postoperatively, even if good analgesia is provided, it is often advisable to administer warmed (39 °C) subcutaneous or intraperitoneal dextrose/saline at the end of surgery to provide some fluid supplementation in the immediate postoperative period. It is preferable to have administered warmed intravenous fluids throughout the operative period but this may not always be practicable. Rabbits should be encouraged to eat as soon as possible after recovery from anaesthesia, as this reduces the incidence of digestive disturbances. Normal gastrointestinal function is more likely if effective postoperative analgesia has been provided but additional measures, such as the use of gastrointestinal motility stimulants (e.g. cisapride or metaclopramide) may also be needed, particularly after gastrointestinal tract surgery.

If animals do not begin to eat and drink within the first few hours after recovery, fluid therapy should be continued and the rabbit hand-fed or fed via an oral or nasogastric tube provided it is fully alert (see Chapter 1).

Analgesia

It is particularly important that good postoperative analgesia is provided, since pain can cause inappetence and prolong the effects of surgery. The analgesics available for use in other companion animal species can be administered safely, although limited information is available for some of the newer NSAIDs. Suggested dose rates are given in Figure 12.7. When major surgery is undertaken (e.g. orthopaedic procedures and mandibular and maxillary surgery as part of dental procedures), the opioid analgesic buprenorphine should be given, either alone or in combination with an NSAID such as carprofen or ketoprofen, since this may provide more effective pain relief than use of either drug alone. Infiltration of the surgical site with a long-acting local anaesthetic, such as bupivacaine, can also be a useful adjunct to the use of systemic analgesics. Less extensive procedures (e.g. uncomplicated ovariohysterectomy or castration) may require only administration of a potent NSAID. Following an initial dose at the time of surgery, an additional dose of an NSAID can be given by mouth 16-24 hours later. In most circumstances, provision of analgesia for 24-48 hours appears sufficient.

There is little detailed information regarding the clinical efficacy of many of these analgesics but many agents have been shown to be safe and effective in laboratory studies. There can be few indications, then, for withholding analgesics. Unfortunately, recent surveys (Capner et al., in press) have indicated that analgesics are used much less frequently in rabbits than in dogs and cats. Aside from concerns as to the safety of analgesic preparations in rabbits (which are largely unfounded), one reason for this lack of analgesic use may be a failure to recognize the signs of pain in this species. Rabbits do not often show obvious signs of pain; in the wild, expressing pain might attract the attention of a predator and so would not be of benefit. Most respond to pain by remaining immobile. They may become apathetic, or agitated, or aggressive when approached or handled and will only vocalize or struggle when in extreme distress. This failure to express overt pain behaviour can result in clinicians assuming that rabbits do not experience as much pain as other species. This is a dangerous and misleading assumption, which can result in rabbits not being given appropriate analgesic therapy. Careful observation of rabbits following surgery allows detection of guarding behaviour, and other signs of pain such as relative immobility, adoption of abnormal posture, moving with an abnormal gait, and teeth-grinding in animals with abdominal pain. If in doubt, it is usually preferable to administer an analgesic. Concerns that analgesic administration predisposes to an animal removing its skin sutures are completely unfounded. In any event, use of a subcuticular suture for wound closure (see Chapter 13) makes this issue irrelevant.

In other species, it is generally recommended that analgesics should be administered preoperatively, as this provides more effective pain relief and also may reduce the dose of anaesthetic required. Experience in rabbits has shown that use of buprenorphine in this way enables the concentration of isoflurane or halothane needed for surgical anaesthesia to be reduced by 0.25-0.5%. Care should be taken when using injectable anaesthetics administered by the subcutaneous or intramuscular routes since in these circumstances it is not possible to adjust the dose of anaesthetic to meet individual requirements, and there are few data available on the potentiating effects of opioids. Until such information is available, it is probably better to administer opioids postoperatively when using injectable anaesthetic agents. When using neuroleptanalgesics, the opioid component will provide analgesia and this can conveniently be partially reversed with buprenorphine or butorphanol. If the latter opioid is used, although it provides better reversal, it has a short duration of action, so either additional doses should be given, or it should be combined with a potent NSAID. When ketamine and medetomidine or xylazine are used, it is often best to reverse anaesthesia partially by administering atipamezole. As mentioned earlier, this reverses the analgesic effect of the alpha$_2$ agonist, so additional analgesic agents must be administered if pain is likely to be present. The author has used carprofen preoperatively (as recommended in other species) but no controlled studies have been undertaken.

Provision of analgesia for 24-48 hours appears sufficient after most procedures, but additional doses of analgesic may be needed after major dental procedures. When providing prolonged analgesia for animals that are to be returned home, the newer potent NSAIDs can be very effective. Administering the drug in tablet form is difficult but these can be crushed and mixed with food. Many rabbits find the oral preparation of meloxicam highly palatable, and this can be a very convenient means for the owner to continue analgesic treatment.

REFERENCES

Aeschbacher G and Webb AI (1993a) Propofol in rabbits. 1. Determination of an induction dose. Laboratory Animal Science, 43, 324-327
Aeschbacher G and Webb AI (1993b) Propofol in rabbits. 2. Long-term anesthesia. Laboratory Animal Science, 43, 328-335
Blake DW, Jover B and McGrath BP (1988) Haemodynamic and heart rate reflex responses to propofol in the rabbit. Comparison with althesin. British Journal of Anaesthesia, 61, 194-199

Capner CA, Lascelles BDX and Waterman-Pearson, AE (In press) A survey of current British veterinary attitudes to peri-operative analgesia. *Veterinary Record*

Clarke KW and Hall LW (1990) A survey of anaesthesia in small animal practice: AVA/BSAVA report. *Journal of the Association of Veterinary Anaesthetists*, **17**, 4-10

Flecknell PA, Cruz IJ, Liles JH and Whelan G (1996) Induction of anaesthesia with halothane and isoflurane in the rabbit: a comparison of the use of a face-mask or an anaesthetic chamber. *Laboratory Animals* **30**, 67-74

Flecknell PA, John M, Mitchell M, Shurey C and Simpkins S (1983) Neuroleptanalgesia in the rabbit. *Laboratory Animals*, **17**, 104-109

Flecknell PA and Liles JH (1990) Assessment of the analgesic action of opioid agonist–antagonists in the rabbit. *Journal of the Association of Veterinary Anaesthetists* **17**, 24-29

Flecknell PA and Waterman-Pearson A (in press) *Pain Management in Animals*. Harcourt-Brace, London

Glen JB (1980) Animal studies of the anaesthetic activity of ICI 35 868. *British Journal of Anaesthesia*, **52,** 731-741

Green CJ, Halsey MJ, Precious S and Simpkin S (1978) Alphaxolone-alphadolone anaesthesia in laboratory animals. *Laboratory Animals*, **12,** 85-89

Ko JCH, Thurmon JC, Tranquilli, WJ, Benson GJ and Olson WA (1992) A comparison of medetomidine–propofol and medetomidine–midazolam–propofol anesthesia in rabbits. *Laboratory Animal Science*, **42**, 503-507.

Lipman NS, Marini RP and Flecknell PA (1997) Anesthesia and analgesia in rabbits. In: *Anesthesia and Analgesia in Laboratory Animals*, ed. DF Kohn *et al*. Academic Press, New York

Peeters ME, Gil D, Teske E, Eyzenbach V, Van De Brom W E, Lumeij J T and De Vries HW (1988) Four methods for general anaesthesia in the rabbit: a comparative study. *Laboratory Animals*, **22**, 355-360

CHAPTER THIRTEEN

Surgical Procedures and Dental Disorders

Sharon Redrobe

GENERAL CONSIDERATIONS FOR SURGERY

A basic knowledge of general surgical techniques and procedures is assumed. This chapter will address common surgical procedures in the rabbit and provide guidance on the surgical approach. Only the relevant surgical anatomy will be included in this chapter.

Preoperative examination
All animals should have a thorough clinical examination prior to surgery. Preoperative blood work including biochemistry, clotting times and haematology may be indicated in individual cases.

Pain management
Good perioperative care, especially with regard to pain management, is vital for the success of the procedure (see Chapter 12). Rabbits in pain may become anorexic and develop ileus, which may be fatal.

Food and water
If the animal is anorexic, nutritional support should be given to prevent hepatic lipidosis. The food and water intake should be monitored pre- and postoperatively, together with the animal's bodyweight.

Preoperative fasting is not required as rabbits cannot vomit. However, prior to abdominal surgery food may be withheld for 6–12 hours to reduce the volume of the gastrointestinal tract. It is not possible to produce a completely empty gastrointestinal tract even after a 24-hour fast in the rabbit.

Body temperature
During anaesthesia, the rabbit patient should be placed on a heat pad and the body temperature monitored. The body temperature of the anaesthetized patient can fall rapidly without supplementary heat, especially when the abdomen is opened. This hypothermia can prove fatal.

Positioning
Breathing may be compromised in the dorsally recumbent rabbit as the weight of the relatively large abdomen presses on the small thorax. This fact is especially relevant in obese rabbits. The head and thorax should therefore be elevated to reduce respiratory compromise.

Asepsis
Aseptic technique is required for all surgical procedures in rabbits, as for other animals. The thick, dense fur of rabbits may easily clog clipper blades, and clippers or scissors easily lacerate the thin skin. Hair removal cream may therefore be used as an alternative to avoid such skin trauma. The use of depilatory cream additionally allows the hair to be removed easily in the conscious rabbit before the induction of anaesthesia, so reducing anaesthetic time. A patch test should be performed prior to applying the cream to large areas to assess any adverse skin reaction to the depilatory cream.

After hair removal, the skin is aseptically prepared in the routine manner. The excessive use of alcohol-based skin antiseptics should be avoided to prevent chilling and predisposing the animal towards hypothermia.

Instrumentation
Magnification is useful to improve visualization at the surgical site. Binocular loupes or an operating microscope may be used.

Either conventional small or microsurgical instruments may be required for rabbit surgery, depending upon the size of the animal and the surgical technique under consideration. It is useful to prepare a small surgery pack supplied with small or special microsurgical instruments, small (or cut down) gauzes and appropriately sized drapes. Clear plastic drapes are useful in rabbit surgery, as they are lightweight and allow visualization of the animal, facilitating intraoperative monitoring.

The placement of an intravenous or intraosseous catheter will assist in the perioperative administration of drugs and fluids (see Chapters 1 and 12).

Blood loss
Limiting blood loss is important in smaller patients. On average, the rabbit has a blood volume of 57 ml/kg bodyweight. Loss of 15–20% will result in tachycardia and arterial constriction, compromising the blood supply to the skin and gastrointestinal tract. An acute loss of 25% will prove fatal. For a 2 kg

rabbit, the amounts are approximately 18 ml and 26 ml of blood loss.

Limiting tissue damage

Intraoperatively, all tissues should be handled gently to limit postoperative inflammation and subsequent self-trauma. The use of radio- or electrosurgical equipment provides accurate haemostasis with minimal tissue damage.

Rabbits are prone to developing ileus and adhesions following abdominal surgery. Handling of the gastrointestinal tract should be minimal and gentle. The abdominal viscera should be frequently moistened with sterile saline to prevent desiccation that may predispose to adhesion formation and ileus. Abdominal lavage should be performed prior to closure of the abdomen to ensure the removal of blood clots. Calcium channel blockers e.g. verapamil (200 μg/kg orally every 8 hours for 9 doses), have been used experimentally to reduce the formation of adhesions. Gastrointestinal tract motility enhancers, e.g. metoclopramide may be injected directly into the affected intestines if ileus is detected intraoperatively, or be administered postoperatively to promote gut function, e.g. oral cisapride.

Suture materials and patterns

Rabbits readily produce a caseous suppurative response to foreign bodies and have a high tendency to form adhesions. It is important to consider these points when choosing suitable suture material or alternatives for rabbit surgery.

The use of catgut is not recommended in rabbits. The absorbable polymers that rely upon hydrolytic degradation should be used as they are less reactive and form weaker adhesions than catgut. Metal clips for vessel ligation and skin sutures form minimal adhesions and are useful to reduce surgical time. Ligature clips are less likely to tear friable vessels than nylon ligatures.

Rabbits are fastidious groomers, and so may easily remove skin sutures. The use of the intradermal or subcuticular skin suture pattern enables good apposition without external sutures. The subcuticular suture is tied using a hidden knot, the 'Aberdeen knot', to prevent further access to the suture material (Figure 13.1).

Cyanoacrylic tissue adhesive can be used to close skin that is not under tension, or to support skin sutures, although some rabbits will find the glue a focus to begin chewing. Skin staples can be used in the skin and are not easily removed by rabbits.

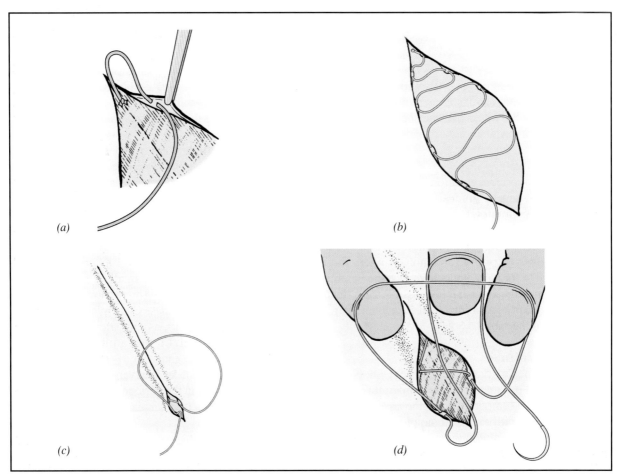

(a)

(b)

(c)

(d)

Figure 13.1: *Subcuticular suture anchored with an 'Aberdeen knot'. (a) Anchoring the suture in the thing subcuticular layer is difficult; it is therefore preferable to place the first knot in the muscle layer. (b) The suture is then run in a continuous pattern in the subcuticular tissue. (c) Conventional anchoring techniques require a final loop to be tied to the long end of the suture. (d) To tie an 'Aberdeen knot', a loop of suture is drawn through the loop formed by the last part of the continuous suture. Reproduced from Flecknell (1998) with permission of* In Practice. ▶

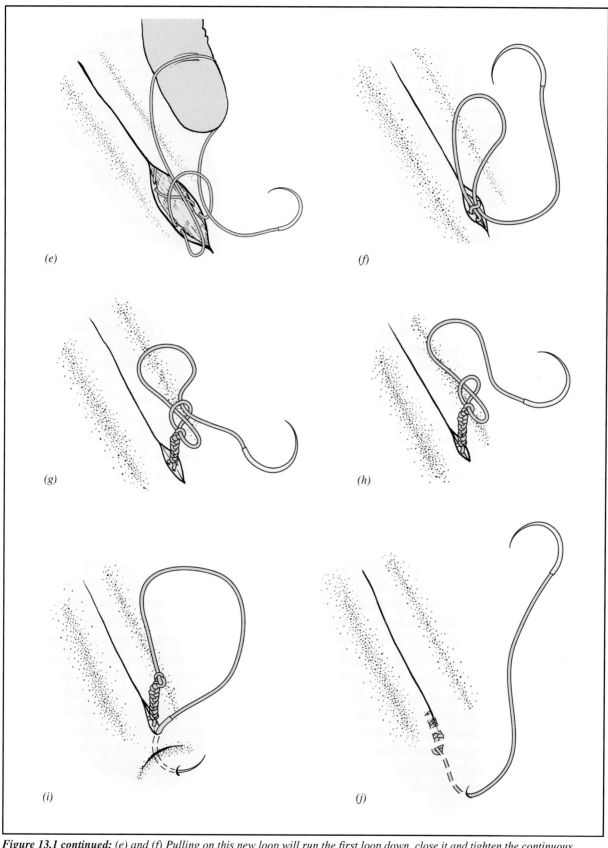

Figure 13.1 continued: (e) and (f) Pulling on this new loop will run the first loop down, close it and tighten the continuous suture. This process is repeated six or seven times, each time forming a new loop by drawing the long end of the suture through the existing loop. (g) Pulling on the new loop runs a knot down on to the suture. (h) The needle is then passed through the last loop and pulled tight to lock the run of knots. (i) The needle is introduced into the end of the wound between the skin and muscle layers and brought out a short distance from the wound edge. (j) Pulling on the suture draws the row of knots under the skin, burying them completely. The suture is cut close to the skin so that the cut end retracts under the skin. Reproduced from Flecknell (1998) with permission of In Practice.

SOFT TISSUE SURGERY TECHNIQUES

Urogenital surgery

Ovariohysterectomy

Indications:

- Uterine adenocarcinoma
- Uterine aneurysm
- Pyometra
- Unwanted pregnancy
- Pseudopregnancy
- Ovarian neoplasia
- Behavioural modification in the management of aggression, sexual behaviour and territorial marking.

Radiography of the thorax should be performed prior to surgery to investigate the presence of pulmonary metastases if uterine adenocarcinoma is suspected. Prophylactic ovariohysterectomy is usually performed between the ages of 4 months and 2 years.

Relevant anatomy: The rabbit possesses a bicornate uterus, each horn leading to a separate cervix (see Chapter 6). There is no uterine body. The uterus lies in the caudal abdomen, dorsal to the urinary bladder.

The mesometrium is a primary fat storage site in the rabbit, making visualization and ligation of the vessels difficult. In younger animals, the amount of fat is small, but in older animals, there may be very extensive deposits. When presented with an obviously obese animal, it may be advisable to encourage a weight reduction programme before elective surgery.

The ovarian ligaments are relatively long so exteriorization of the ovaries, horns and cervices is therefore easily achieved. Accessory vessels are often present in a variable number and not arranged symmetrically in the broad ligament. The uterus becomes engorged in the pregnant or pseudopregnant female, making the associated blood vessels more friable.

The urethra opens into the proximal end of the vaginal vestibule. Manual expression of the bladder while the rabbit is in dorsal recumbency should be avoided as this practice increases the risk of filling the vestibule with urine. The pooled urine may serve as a source of contamination during uterine surgery.

Surgical technique: The ovariohysterectomy procedure is illustrated in Figure 13.2.

1. The anaesthetized rabbit is restrained in dorsal recumbency with the hind limbs restrained in extension.
2. A 2–3 cm midline skin incision is made midway between the umbilicus and the cranial rim of the pelvis.

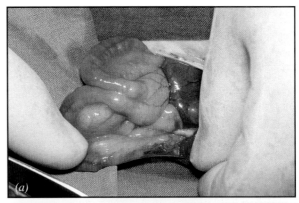
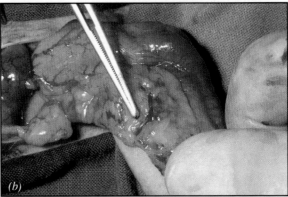
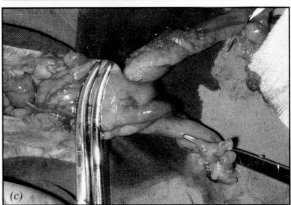
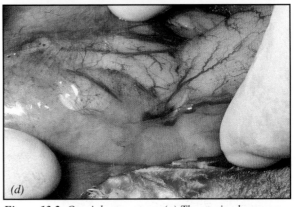

Figure 13.2: *Ovariohysterectomy.(a) The uterine horns are exposed, the ovarian vessels are clamped and ligated, and the ovarian ligament is divided. (b) Care must be taken to locate and avoid vessels embedded in the fat depots in the broad ligament. (c) The uterus is clamped and the vessels ligated before removal of the uterine body. (d) The uterus is highly mobile, but should not be retracted too much, as clamping lower down on the cervix can damage vessels supplying the bladder.*

3. The linea alba is identified, the abdominal muscles elevated and a guarded scalpel or blunt-ended scissors used to incise the body wall. Care is taken to avoid the thin-walled caecum and urinary bladder that are often pressing against the abdominal wall in this position.
4. The uterus is pink and flat compared to the darker and rounder small intestine; it is located and exteriorized.
5. The ovaries are located at the end of each horn. Care should be taken to ensure the ovary is removed with the uterine horn. The ovary is often hidden in fat and difficult to visualize. It may be palpated as a small pea-shape within the associated fat.
6. The ovarian pedicle is located, adipose tissue dissected away and the pedicle ligated using a transfixing suture. Caution should be taken when applying haemostats to the pedicle as the vessels are easily lacerated. There is not often room to employ the three-clamp technique as in the bitch. The ovarian ligaments should not be pulled as they are easily torn, and care should be taken as suture material may lacerate engorged vessels. The use of electro- or radiocautery greatly assists the surgeon in achieving haemostasis of these vessels. The use of metal vascular clips reduces the risk of laceration and can considerably reduce the surgical time required for this procedure.
7. The stumps should be inspected for bleeding before they are released into the abdomen. The vessels of the mesometrium are identified and ligated/coagulated down to the level of the cervices. There are variable numbers of accessory vessels supplying the uterus: these vessels are often hidden in the fat associated with the broad ligament, are more friable than in the dog or cat and are easy torn on dissection of the fat. The vessels must be identified and ligated individually.
8. The uterus may be removed proximal or caudal to the cervices. It is preferable to excise the uterus caudal to the cervices for the treatment of uterine neoplasia to ensure all the uterine tissue is removed. If the uterus is removed caudal to the cervix, the reproductive tract must be sealed securely to prevent urine leakage into the abdomen.
9. The ureters should be identified to avoid their accidental ligation. Care should be taken that the blood vessels supplying the bladder are not accidentally clamped. This can occur if the uterine clamp is placed too far caudally.
10. The uterus or distal vagina is double ligated with transfixing sutures. The ovarian and cervical stumps are checked for haemorrhage prior to closure of the abdomen.
11. The author prefers to use simple interrupted sutures for the closure of the abdominal wall. The subcuticular tissue is closed using a simple continuous pattern. The skin is closed using a hidden subcuticular technique or skin staples.
12. It may be beneficial to administer one dose of metoclopramide postoperatively to prevent ileus. This is especially important in cases of prolonged surgery or manipulation of the gastrointestinal tract.

Caesarian section

Indications: These are:

- Dystocia
- Uterine inertia.

Abdominal palpation, radiography and ultrasonography may be used in the detection of pregnancy/retained fetus(es) and the assessment of the viability of the fetus(es).

Rabbits usually produce the litter of kittens overnight and the delivery of the whole litter occurs in less than one hour. An interval between delivery of the kits in excess of one hour, straining, palpation of remaining kitten(s), with or without straining at full term, or after the delivery of some kittens, are indications for further investigation. Medical therapy (calcium, oxytocin) may be used initially if non-obstructive dystocia or uterine inertia is diagnosed. The rabbit should be stabilized prior to surgery.

Relevant anatomy: See ovariohysterectomy.

Surgical technique:

1. The anaesthetized rabbit is restrained in dorsal recumbency with the hindlimbs in extension. The rabbit is held in a position with the head elevated at 10–20 degrees to reduce the pressure of the abdominal contents on the thorax. Surgical speed is important to avoid fetal asphyxia.
2. The ventral abdomen from the xiphoid sternum to pubis is aseptically prepared.
3. A midline abdominal incision from xiphoid to pubis is made in a routine manner, avoiding the enlarged mammary glands and associated blood vessels.
4. The abdomen is packed with saline-moistened swabs to limit abdominal contamination.
5. The gravid uterus is located.
6. The fetus closest to the cervices is removed first. The uterine incision is made over the fetal limb, taking great care to avoid lacerating the fetus. The placenta is removed with the fetus, if possible.
7. The umbilicus is clamped and the delivered kitten rubbed vigorously with a towel to dry it and stimulate breathing. Fetal membranes and fluid are cleared from the mouth and nostrils and doxapram can be given orally to stimulate breathing if required.

8. If uterine contractions are not seen prior to abdominal closure, oxytocin (1–2 IU/kg i.m. or i.v.) may be administered to stimulate uterine contractions and milk production.
9. The uterine wall is closed using a double layer inverting suture pattern.
10. The abdomen is lavaged with isotonic saline warmed to room temperature prior to routine closure of the abdomen.

Postoperative considerations: Oxytocin may be repeated 2–4 hours postoperatively to limit uterine haemorrhage and stimulate milk production. Supportive care for the dam is provided as required.

Castration

Relevant anatomy: The testes are located in thin-walled scrotal sacs in the inguinal area and are easily visualized externally in the sexually mature male. Rabbits possess an open inguinal ring that allows the testes to be withdrawn into the abdomen. A careful preoperative examination should be undertaken to establish that both testes have descended into the scrotal sacs. If the plane of anaesthesia is too light, the testis may be retracted during preparation of the skin or on making the first incision.

Herniation of the abdominal contents through the inguinal canal after castration is rare, due to the presence of an epididymal fat pad located over the internal inguinal ring. Nevertheless, closed castration is recommended to decrease the risk of herniation.

Indications:

• Prevention of breeding
• Removal of retained testes
• Testicular neoplasia
• Severe testicular trauma
• Orchitis or epididymitis non-responsive to medical therapy
• Behavioural problems e.g. urine marking, territorial aggression.

Prophylactic castration is generally performed in the rabbit over 4 months of age. Neutering is required if two or more male rabbits are to be housed together, to reduce aggression.

Surgical technique:

1. The rabbit is anaesthetized and restrained in dorsal recumbency with the hind limbs restrained caudally.
2. The scrotal sacs, caudal abdomen and medial thighs are aseptically prepared. Great care must be taken to avoid lacerating the thin skin of the scrotal sacs with clippers.

3. The thin skin of the scrotum is incised (Figure 13.3a). The vaginal tunic is left intact in order to perform a closed castration. The skin is tightly adherent to the testis and is stripped away using blunt dissection to exteriorize the testis (Figure 13.3b).
4. The proper ligament is bluntly dissected to free the testis.
5. In older or obese males, the cord contains a large amount of fat, making identification of the cord structures difficult. The junction between the testis and the fatty cord can be identified by palpation prior to suture placement. The vessels within the cord are more friable than in the dog or cat and great care must be used in applying haemostats prior to suture placement. The cord is double ligated using a transfixing ligature. A transfixing ligature is required to ensure the blood vessels in the fatty cord are adequately ligated (Figure 13.3c).

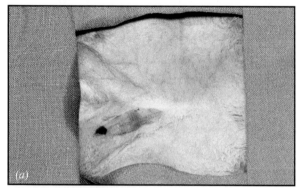

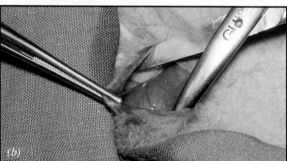

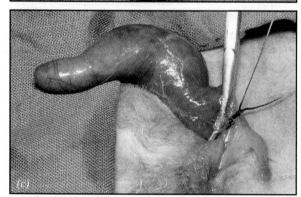

Figure 13.3: Castration. (a) A skin incision is made on the anterior aspect of the scrotum, to expose the tunic. (b) The testis is dissected free, leaving the tunic intact. (c) The cord is clamped and ligated with one or two transfixing ligatures, and the testis removed.

6. Either a second skin incision can be made or the remaining testis is dissected free via the initial incision, taking care to avoid trauma to the penis.
7. Closure of the inguinal rings is not required if a closed castration technique is performed. An extra subcutaneous layer of sutures may be placed before the skin is closed as an added precaution as rabbits have a higher incidence of self-trauma postoperatively than cats and dogs.
8. The scrotal skin may be closed using a subcuticular suture pattern or cyanoacrylate glue.

Postoperative considerations: Scrotal haematomas may form in the postoperative period. This may be due to self-trauma, excessive exercise on recovery, ligature slippage, or seepage from the ligated stump if the vessels of the cord were friable and damaged during the surgery. It is wise, therefore, to ensure:

- The use of transfixing sutures and atraumatic closure of the scrotal skin
- Adequate use of non-steroidal anti-inflammatory drugs (NSAID) or other analgesic drugs
- Limitation of the rabbit to cage rest overnight
- Close observation of the animal for several hours postoperatively.

Retained testis or testes

Relevant anatomy: The ductus deferens courses within the abdomen from the abdominal inguinal ring to the prostatic urethra (see Chapter 6). Each ductus courses caudally and medially around the ipsilateral ureter at the level of the lateral ligament of the bladder. The ureter normally lies dorsal to the ductus. The retained testis may be located on the route between the caudal aspect of the kidney to the cranial aspect of the scrotum.

Indication: Testicular retention. Complete agenesis of a testis is extremely rare, and so a testis that is not external has almost certainly been retained. Retained testes are predisposed to malignant transformation e.g. seminoma and Sertoli cell tumour, and so exploratory surgery and removal is indicated.

Surgical technique:

1. The scrotal sacs and inguinal area are gently explored during the preoperative examination to check for the presence of the undescended testis. A nervous rabbit may retract the testis into the abdomen on physical examination. The examination is repeated when the animal is under a general anaesthetic.
2. If no testis is located, a routine midline incision is made into the abdomen (see ovariohysterectomy technique).

3. The area cranial to the scrotum to caudal to the kidney is explored. The retained testis is often readily visible as a mobile, small testis in the mid abdomen. If not readily visible, the abdominal wall is palpated to the level of the inguinal ring or the incision is extended caudally and the ductus deferens identified at the level of the ureter and followed proximally to the testis.
4. The associated vessels are double ligated and the testis removed.
5. The abdomen is closed routinely.

Cystocentesis

Indication: For the collection of a urine sample for analysis in the investigation of urine scald, urolithiasis and cystitis.

Relevant anatomy: The bladder is situated in the mid-caudal abdomen just cranial to the pubic region.

Technique:

1. The rabbit is restrained in dorsal recumbency either conscious, under sedation or with a full general anaesthetic.
2. The area cranial and midline to the pubic region is clipped and aseptically prepared.
3. The bladder is located by palpation and stabilized between fingers and thumb.
4. A 23–25G needle with a 2 ml or 5 ml syringe attached is advanced craniocaudally into the bladder and urine aspirated.

Cystotomy

Indications:

- Urine scald
- Urolithiasis
- Neoplasia.

Urinalysis, urine culture, plain radiography, contrast cystography, ultrasonography of the bladder and kidneys, and an evaluation of renal function should be conducted prior to surgery.

If urolithiasis is diagnosed, the owner should be warned about the possibility of recurrence of this condition. Although the radiographic finding of 'sand' in the urinary bladder (see Figure 6.4) can be an incidental one in clinically healthy rabbits, it is associated with urine scald in some rabbits. This 'sand' (usually calcium carbonate crystals) can be removed by flushing the bladder with warm saline via a urethral catheter. If this technique is not successful, surgery to lavage the bladder thoroughly may be indicated.

Relevant anatomy: The urinary bladder may rupture when grossly distended or handled roughly during surgery. The bladder wall may be grossly thickened to many times the normal thickness if irritated or infected e.g. by urolithiasis or cystitis.

Surgical technique:

1. The rabbit is prepared for abdominal surgery in a routine manner.
2. The incision is made in the midline through the linea alba from the pubis to the umbilicus. The abdomen is packed with moist swabs.
3. The bladder is drained by cystocentesis if required.
4. Stay sutures are placed in the bladder at the cranial and caudal edge of the proposed incision.
5. The bladder is incised and explored. Uroliths or 'sand' are removed.
6. The bladder is lavaged with a large volume of isotonic saline warmed to body temperature. A catheter is passed into the urethra, which is then flushed to dislodge any urethral calculi and ensure patency.
7. Biopsies of the bladder wall are taken in cases of suspected neoplasia.
8. The bladder is closed using a single layer inverting suture pattern that does not penetrate into the lumen of the bladder. Closure of the abdomen is routine.

Postoperative considerations: Analgesia should be given to reduce the incidence of urethral spasm. If the rabbit does not urinate freely within a few hours postoperatively, a urinary catheter is placed for up to 3 days. Water should be freely available; a fruit flavouring may be added to the water to increase intake. The calcium content of the diet may be reduced to decrease the formation of calcium carbonate crystals in the urine.

Gastrointestinal surgery

Gastrotomy

Relevant anatomy: Rabbits cannot vomit, so ingested material that is unable to pass out of the pylorus will lead to blockage. Gastric foreign bodies are often associated with gastric ulceration that may rapidly progress to perforation if the condition is not treated quickly.

Indications:

- Trichobezoars (hairballs)
- Foreign body impaction
- Neoplasia.

Clinical signs include: acute-onset abdominal pain; gastric dilation due to gastric or duodenal obstruction; bloat; intermittent abdominal pain; and intermittent diarrhoea or constipation.

Diagnostic approach: The animal should be stabilized prior to surgery using analgesia, parenteral fluids and short-acting corticosteroids. If gastric bloat is present, decompression by passing a naso- or orogastric tube should be attempted.

Radiography may reveal the foreign body or disorder of the gastrointestinal tract. Contrast radiography will aid in differentiating some masses. The use of barium is to be avoided in cases where gastrointestinal tract rupture is suspected.

Trichobezoars (hairballs) usually require medical, not surgical, management including aggressive fluid therapy, force feeding (syringe feeding or via a nasogastric tube) and a high fibre diet (see Chapter 5). The patient will require a positive energy balance and correction of electrolyte imbalances. Hepatic lipidosis, acidosis and ketosis may all feature in the clinical syndrome. Ulceration of the stomach can occur associated with gastric immotility, foreign body or trichobezoar. Specific treatment for ulceration should be given. Ulceration may progress to perforation and peritonitis, which carries a poor prognosis. Drugs such as cisapride, metoclopramide, histamine blockers and analgesics may all be used in the medical treatment of this condition.

The clinician should also consider the possible underlying causes of ileus e.g. pain, dysbiosis, adhesions, and dysautonomia. If the foreign body within the stomach does not move within 3 or 4 days and there is no associated ileus present then the animal may be considered a surgical candidate once stabilized.

Surgical technique:

1. The rabbit is shaved from pubis to mid-thorax and placed in dorsal recumbency.
2. A midline incision is made. Care should be taken not to damage the caecum and stomach, as these organs are thin walled when distended.
3. The abdomen is explored for other lesions. A gastric or duodenal obstruction is often associated with a necrotic duodenum that will require resection at laparotomy. A liver biopsy is indicated if it appears abnormal; the biopsy method is routine.
4. Stay sutures are placed in the stomach and the greater curvature elevated. The abdomen is packed with moist swabs to prevent abdominal contamination.
5. The gastric incision is made in the avascular area between the greater and lesser curvatures.
6. The foreign body or impaction is identified and removed.

7. The stomach is lavaged and the lumen examined. The patency of the pylorus is ascertained.
8. The stomach is closed in a two-layer inverting suture pattern using 3/0 synthetic monofilament. The abdomen is lavaged thoroughly with isotonic fluids warmed to body temperature.

Postoperative considerations: Supportive postoperative therapy (e.g. analgesia, gut motility enhancers, nutritional and hepatic support) is required to promote a rapid recovery.

Intestinal resection, anastomoses and enterotomy

Indications:

• Intestinal foreign body
• Caecoliths
• Caecophytobezoars
• Metastatic uterine adenocarcinomas
• Severe bite wound trauma
• Iatrogenic intraoperative trauma
• Neoplasia
• Rectal polyps and metastases.

A gastric or duodenal obstruction is often associated with a necrotic duodenum that will require resection at laparotomy. Clinical signs include: acute-onset abdominal pain; gastric dilation due to gastric or duodenal obstruction; bloat: intermittent abdominal pain; and intermittent diarrhoea or constipation.

Relevant anatomy: The serous membrane of the caecum is thin and easily torn when handled or sutured. The rabbit's intestine has a small lumen and a relatively thick visceral wall. The caudal end of the ileum is modified to form a round, muscular enlargement termed the sacculus rotundus. Material is directed to the caecum or colon from this region. The sacculus rotundus is a common site for foreign body impaction. Other common sites include stomach, ileocaecocolic junction, caecum and colon.

Surgical technique: The basic principles are as for the dog and cat. Preparation of the animal is as for gastrotomy. The abdomen is opened routinely. The entire contents of the gastrointestinal tract should be carefully examined; it is important to preserve the blood supply and lumen diameter. The gastrointestinal tract should be handled gently to prevent shock and postoperative ileus.

Small intestine

1. The mesenteric and arcade vessels are ligated and clamps applied to the bowel as with other species.
2. The intestines are transected at an acute angle to increase lumen diameter following anastomosis.

3. The gut is closed using 4/0 or 6/0 monofilament suture material. A linear foreign body may lead to bowel plication and intussusception and require multiple enterotomy sites. Longitudinal incisions are generally closed using a transverse closure method to increase lumen diameter.

Large intestine

1. The bowel should be incised at an acute angle with longitudinal incisions, and transverse closures utilized to increase diameter.
2. The anastomosis is performed using interrupted suture patterns of opposition or crushing types in the colon. An inverting suture technique should be used in the caecum. 4/0 or 6/0 monofilament suture material should be used. The omentum may be used to reinforce the suture line.

Prior to closure the abdomen should be lavaged with copious amounts of isotonic saline warmed to body temperature and suction used to remove excess fluid. A swab of free abdominal contents in the case of bowel rupture should be submitted for aerobic and anaerobic culture and appropriate antibiotics given.

Anorectal papilloma removal

Indications:

• Bleeding from the anus
• Prolapse
• Constipation and discomfort.

Relevant anatomy
Anorectal papillomas resemble fungating masses at the anorectal junction. They are usually benign. They may protrude from the anus once they are large enough; they tend to be friable and bleed easily. Papillomas may be attached by a stalk or a broad base.

Surgical technique:
The animal should be under a general anaesthetic and restrained in dorsal recumbency with the pelvis elevated. A speculum is inserted into the anus and/or stay sutures applied. Sharp dissection, electro- or radiosurgery is used to excise the mass. Adequate resection requires good visualization. All the abnormal tissue must be removed to prevent recurrence.

ORTHOPAEDIC TECHNIQUES

In general, techniques applicable to the dog and cat are used in the rabbit. The cortices of rabbit bones are hard and brittle compared to those of the cat. The bones of the rabbit comprise only 8% of the total bodyweight, compared to 13% in the cat. The bones of rabbits do, however, heal well following routine orthopaedic procedures. Rabbits may chew at bandages and so an extra 'chew' layer or tags may be added to the bandage to distract the rabbit. Elizabethan collars may be used but are not tolerated by some rabbits.

Fracture fixation

Fractures tend to be comminuted and are often open and contaminated on initial presentation. Rabbits readily develop osteomyelitis in these situations, and attention should be given to cleaning the fracture site, maintaining asepsis during surgery, and the provision of postoperative antibiotics.

The small size of rabbit bones often precludes the use of standard orthopaedic plates. Small plates manufactured for human finger fixation may be used. Closed pin techniques may also be employed. The intramedullary pin should occupy approximately 70% of the medullary cavity. Also, the small size of many rabbits suggests the use of Kirschner wires. Cerclage wires may be used in combination with intramedullary pins as in other species.

An external fixator may be applied to fractures of the limbs (Figure 13.4). This method of fixation allows postoperative weight-bearing, does not require additional bandaging, provides rigid stability and involves minimal soft tissue damage. Threaded pins are rarely necessary due to the small bone size and rapid bone healing time of rabbits.

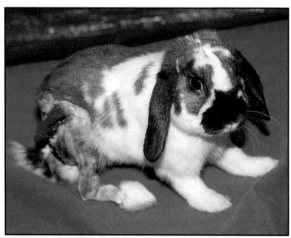

Figure 13.4: *Rabbit with external uniplanar fixator on the femur.*

Bone cement, cast material shaped into a tube or acrylics may be used as fixator bars to produce the small size and lightweight fixators required. The fixator pin diameter should not exceed 20% of the bone diameter, as in other animals. Kirschner wires or hypodermic needles may be used as fixator pins in small rabbits.

Three pins per segment should be applied if space permits. The fixator pins may be placed percutaneously in areas of limited soft tissue coverage for the

fixation of simple distal limb fractures. Stab incisions in the skin are made to allow pin insertion with minimal soft tissue trauma.

Highly comminuted fractures or fractures requiring debridement should be fixed using an open technique after appropriate cleansing and fracture reduction. The animal should be checked every 2 weeks for pin loosening, tract infection and fracture stability. Pin removal is generally at 6 weeks postoperatively, based upon clinical and radiographic examination.

Padded bandages and split casts may be used. The use of lightweight cast material is recommended to avoid excessive weight on the limb.

Limb amputation

Indications

- Irreparable damage to the limb
- Salvage treatment for severe pododermatitis, osteomyelitis, neoplasia
- Salvage surgery for fractures based on financial considerations (if amputation is cheaper than fixation techniques).

Periosteal proliferation of the tarsometatarsus has been associated with an intrapulmonary mass in a rabbit (DeSanto, 1997); therefore, thoracic radiographs should be taken in the investigation of such lesions prior to surgery.

Surgical technique

The muscles are removed from the distal limb by incising through the tendons. The bone is cut with a high-speed saw. Rabbit bones readily shatter and so crushing bone cutters should not be used. The end of the bone is plugged with bone wax. The bony stump should be cushioned with a muscle belly.

Fore limb: Amputation should be performed at the level of the shoulder in a similar technique to that used in dogs and cats (Figure 13.5). The scapula may be removed to achieve a more cosmetic result.

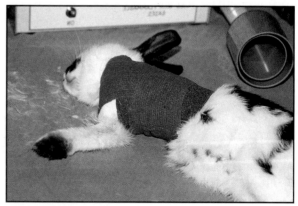

Figure 13.5: *Appearance of rabbit after limb amputation.*

Hind limb: The heavy muscle of the limb requires amputation through the proximal third of the femur. More proximal trauma indicates amputation via disarticulation of the coxofemoral joint. The stump is left to protect the perineal area and genitalia.

Postoperative considerations

Rabbits generally adapt well to only having three legs, even following hind limb amputations. Possible complications include the formation of a seroma and penetration of the bone through the skin in very active animals if amputation was made through the limb bone rather than via disarticulation of a joint.

Correction of elbow luxation

Indication

There is non-weight-bearing lameness of forelimb and swelling of elbow joint, with a history of trauma.

Radiography will demonstrate the elbow luxation; the radius and ulna are usually caudally displaced.

Surgical technique

Closed reduction may be achieved with the rabbit under sedation or general anaesthesia and the limb is then bandaged in extension. This may be sufficient to correct the luxation.

Alternatively, the joint may be fixed using a transarticular pin and splint bandaging. The pin is removed after 3 weeks and the splint maintained for a further 3 weeks. Transarticular external fixators may also be used. Surgical technique is routine.

Bulla osteotomy

Indications

- Neoplasia of the associated area
- Severe refractory chronic otitis media (bacterial or fungal) indicated by head tilt, opisthotonus, horizontal nystagmus and anorexia.

Radiography should be performed to assess the extent of the middle ear disease. Five views are required: dorsoventral; open mouth craniocaudal; lateral; and two oblique views to view the bullae individually. An increase in the density of the bullae may indicate the presence of fluid, exudate, debris, neoplasia or osteomyelitis.

Relevant anatomy

The osseous bulla is part of the middle ear, together with the Eustachian tube, the ossicles and the tympanic membrane. The bone of the osseous bulla is thinnest at the ventral, medial and caudal parts and thicker in the rostral and lateral areas. The facial nerve and sympathetic trunk pass through the middle ear. Rabbits, unlike dogs, do not tend to develop ceruminous gland hyperplasia in response to chronic otitis; therefore, lateral wall resection or canal ablation techniques are rarely required.

Surgical technique

A ventral rather than lateral approach is preferred to achieve good surgical exposure. This provides access to both bullae without patient repositioning being required, ease of preservation of the facial nerve; it also allows ventral drainage postoperatively.

1. The anaesthetized rabbit is restrained in dorsal recumbency with the neck extended.
2. A 4–5 cm incision is made at a point midway between the angle of the mandible and the wings of the atlas.
3. The digastricus muscle is bluntly dissected from the hypoglossal and styloglossal muscles. The hypoglossal nerve is located on the lateral aspect of the hypoglossal muscle and should be avoided.
4. Blunt dissection is directed on to the bulla. The periosteum is elevated.
5. The small tendon passing over the bulla is noted and the bone incised medial to this where the bone is thinner. A burr or Steinmann pin is used to enter the bulla and rongeurs used to extend the opening. Samples are taken for microbial culture and cytology.
6. The osseous bulla is thoroughly irrigated with saline. The lining is curetted out, taking care to avoid the dorsomedial area where the ossicles and promontory are located, disturbance of which will produce vestibular signs in the rabbit.
7. An ingress–egress drain is inserted into the bulla and exited via stab excisions through the main surgical incision.
8. The volume of the bulla is measured using saline intraoperatively; this is usually approximately 1.5 ml.
9. The muscle and subcutaneous tissues are closed in a routine manner.

Postoperative considerations

One end of the drain is closed; saline or antibiotics are instilled into the bulla, left for a minute and then allowed to drain out. This is repeated immediately two or three times. This procedure is repeated three times per day for 7–10 days. Appropriate systemic antimicrobial therapy may be instigated. The rabbit is radiographed and clinically examined 28 days later.

Postoperative complications

- Facial nerve palsy, indicated by loss of the palpebral reflex, inability to move the facial muscles and exposure keratitis
- Vestibular dysfunction, recognized through head tilt, torticollis, nystagmus or rolling of the whole body

- Horner's syndrome will be seen if the sympathetic trunk has been damaged, and presents as miosis, ptosis and enophthalmos
- Hypoglossal nerve palsy is rarely seen, but may occur if the nerve is damaged during dissection and presents as a transient tongue dysfunction.

MISCELLANEOUS CONDITIONS

Dermoplasty or tail amputation for the treatment of urine scald

Indications

- Obesity
- Dysbiosis
- Urinary tract infection
- Spinal problems.

The underlying problem must first be addressed. This is a salvage procedure and should only be undertaken as a last resort to improve the quality of the rabbit's life. It may be considered if the underlying problem cannot be alleviated (e.g. spinal lesions, arthritis), or if the skin is irreparably damaged and reducing the quality of life.

Relevant anatomy

An obese rabbit may develop a fold of skin and fat that covers the genital area and interferes with the normal urine flow. If the animal is still able to rotate the pelvis sufficiently, a skin fold resection technique may be used successfully to alleviate the scalding. Injured or old animals, or those with a spinal problem, may not be able to rotate the pelvis to direct the stream of urine away from the perineum and legs, and require a more radical technique, such as tail amputation, to prevent urine scalding.

Surgical techniques

Antibiotics and anti-inflammatory drugs should be given to minimize inflammation and infection of the area prior to surgery.

Skin fold resection:

1. The animal is anaesthetized and restrained in dorsal recumbency.
2. Hair is removed from the ventral area and the skin is aseptically prepared. A crescent area of skin cranial to the genital area on the abdomen is marked with a pen. This area must be sufficient to lift the excessive skin away from the genital area. Care is taken to avoid the lateral abdominal vein, lateral to the nipple.
3. The inguinal adipose body is removed.
4. An appropriate area of skin is removed.

5. The incision is closed using a tension-relieving suture pattern.

Tail amputation:

1. The animal is anaesthetized and restrained in ventral recumbency, with the hind legs extended.
2. An area 6–8 cm diameter around the anus and tail is aseptically prepared. A crescent-shaped area of skin is marked, sufficient to direct the anus and urethral opening to a more dorsal position.
3. The crescent incision is made dorsal to the anus beyond the dorsal margin of the external anal sphincter muscle on its ventral curvature to just dorsally to the tail, lateral and ventral to the urethral opening.
4. The coccygeal muscle and lateral ventral sacrocaudal muscle of the coccygeal vertebrae should be identified and incised at their insertions.
5. If the animal is male, the retractor penis muscle should be identified and sometimes requires careful dissection from its origin.
6. The tail is amputated at the third or fourth coccygeal vertebra.
7. The medial sacral artery is ligated.
8. The coccygeal and retractor penis muscles are reattached at the dorsal caudal origin of the semitendinosus muscle using synthetic monofilament suture.
9. The skin is closed routinely in two layers. A vertical mattress suture pattern is used to close and relieve tension on the skin layers.

Enucleation of the eye

Indications

- Lack of response to medical therapy for hypopyon, glaucoma, uveitis, and keratitis
- Corneal perforation
- Intraocular neoplasia
- Retrobulbar neoplasia
- Abscess.

Radiography of the skull should be undertaken to investigate any associated bone pathology. Buphthalmos has been reported associated with an intrathoracic mass, suggesting that thoracic radiography may be indicated in the investigation of ocular protrusion.

Relevant anatomy

Rabbits possess a large orbital venous sinus that surrounds the muscle cone and Harderian gland posterior to the globe. Incision of the sinus can lead to profuse, even fatal, haemorrhage.

Surgical technique

A transconjunctival approach is recommended. The dissection should be made along the surface of the globe in order to avoid accidental incision of the orbital sinus. Once the globe is freed, a haemostatic clip is applied to the optic nerve and associated blood vessels before complete excision. If an associated abscess is present, surgical debridement and copious lavage may be performed to remove the purulent material and abscess capsule. A drain may be placed to allow postoperative drainage and/or lavage.

Removal of abscesses

Indications

Abscessation associated with:

* Bite wounds
* Trauma
* Periodontal disease
* Nasolacrimal duct infection or rupture
* Haematogenous spread of infection.

Rabbit abscesses tend to be thick walled and filled with caseous, purulent material. Common bacteria involved include: *Staphylococcus aureus, Pasteurella multocida, Streptococcus, Fusobacterium, Pseudomonas aeruginosa, Corynyebacterium pyogenes, Escherichia coli* and *Klebsiella*.

Complete surgical resection is required, as parental antibiosis or simple lancing and draining are often unsuccessful. The abscess may be opened and allowed to drain, although a high incidence of recurrence is seen if the abscess and capsule are not completely excised.

Abscesses associated with dental infections are common. They may occur secondary to pulp infection of iatrogenic longitudinal fractures that are caused by teeth clipping. The abscesses tend to consist of mixed bacterial or pure Pasteurella multocida or Staphylococcus aureus infections. Total excision of these abscesses is not possible and therefore a guarded prognosis should be given. If radiography reveals an associated osteomyelitis then the prognosis is grave.

Surgical technique

Associated blood vessels are identified and ligated during resection. Skin flap reconstruction techniques may be required if large areas of skin are removed.

Abscesses associated with the feet or of the face require radiography to investigate any underlying osteomyelitis or bony lesions. In some cases, amputation of the affected limb may be required to provide resolution of the infection.

For dental abscesses, aggressive debridement and curettage should be instigated with extraction of the affected teeth (see below). Destruction or removal of

the abscess capsule is vital to achieve resolution of the abscess. This can be achieved chemically (e.g. by flushing with hydrogen peroxide), mechanically (by dissection), or by using radiosurgery. The surgical site may be left open and irrigated daily or partly closed and a drain inserted. Systemic antibiotics based upon culture and sensitivity results should be instigated. The cavity may be packed with calcium hydroxide or antibiotic-impregnated beads. The addition of lignocaine gel to the paste may aid in analgesia.

Postoperative considerations

Analgesia, antibiosis and nutritional support are provided as required. If osteomyelitis is diagnosed, then radiography repeated at 4-week intervals may be used to assess the condition.

NORMAL DENTITION

The normal dentition of the rabbit is shown in the radiographs in Figure 13.6. The dental formula of the rabbit is:

2 x (I 2/1 C 0/0 PM 3/2 M 3/3).

The total number of teeth is therefore 28. There are no canine teeth. The gap between the incisors and premolars is known as the diastema. The premolars and molars are often grouped together and called the 'cheek' teeth.

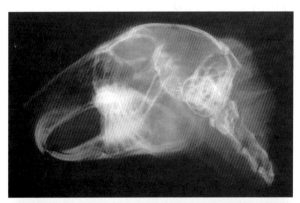
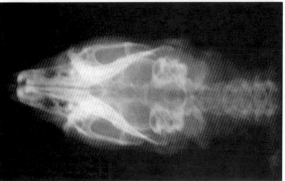

Figure 13.6: *Lateral and dorsoventral radiographs of skull showing normal dental arcade and incisors.*

Rabbits possess aradicular hypsodont teeth, which means that they erupt and grow throughout life and do not have true roots. The incisors grow at a rate of 8–12 cm per year. The continuous growth of the teeth means that the animals can suffer from both primary and secondary problems that may require repeated treatment.

The lips prehend the food, the incisors are used to gnaw and slice the food and the cheek teeth grind the food. The mandible is narrower than the maxilla. Rabbits chew and gnaw by moving the jaws laterally. At rest, the mandibular incisors contact the first and second maxillary incisors. The cheek teeth are out of occlusion when gnawing, so that the incisors alone are in wear. The position of the incisors relative to each other and the fact that the enamel is thicker on the labial surface lead to a faster rate of wear of the lingual side. This produces the characteristic chisel shape of the incisors. When chewing is required, the mandible is retracted to separate the incisors and bring the cheek teeth into occlusion.

THE DENTAL EXAMINATION

A cursory examination may be made in the conscious rabbit using an otoscope or small vaginal speculum intraorally, but such an examination in the conscious rabbit is extremely limited and many lesions will not be detected. A full oral examination to inspect the teeth and soft tissue structures in the mouth requires deep sedation or a full general anaesthetic to abolish chewing movement and allow adequate visualization of the oral cavity. Proprietary oral gags and cheek retractors are available. Alternatively, lengths of bandage hooked over the incisors may be used to open the mouth and allow good visualization with minimal obstruction.

Retraction of the tongue to each side in turn is required to check for spurs that may embed into the base of the tongue. The entire length of the tongue should be examined for signs of laceration or infection. Similarly, the cheeks should be retracted from the dental arcades and examined for evidence of laceration or infection.

The periodontal ligament of each tooth is checked using a blunt probe. The probe is introduced into the gingival sulcus and used to explore around each tooth to check for periodontal pockets, food impaction, plaque, pus and areas of inflammation. Bleeding after probing is a sign of inflammation. Each tooth is checked for excessive mobility.

The results of the dental examination should be recorded on a dental chart for accurate comparison with subsequent examinations. Radiography will aid in the location of spurs and in the assessment of tooth and jaw pathology.

DENTAL DISORDERS

General malocclusion

This is the commonest cause of dental disease in the rabbit. There are six main aetiologies, although in some cases more than one factor may contribute to the clinical problem:

- Congenital deformity, e.g. mandibular prognathism in some dwarf breeds. Mandibular prognathism is thought to be caused by an autosomal recessive trait with incomplete penetrance of 81%. The clinical problem first presents at 8–10 weeks of age, although some animals are presented initially at 12–18 months old
- Dietary problems, e.g. calcium deficiency leading to alveolar bone resorption and tooth loosening, or concentrate-based diet leading to lack of wear and tooth overgrowth
- Trauma to the teeth, e.g. gnawing on bars, falling from a height, tooth clipping
- Fracture of the mandibular ramus presenting as deviation of mandibular incisors to affected side (may occur iatrogenically during extraction). Other skull or jaw fractures are less common
- Infection of tooth roots in the jaw; pulp infection
- Neoplasia affecting the normal anatomy of the jaw, and consequently the dental occlusion.

Incisor malocclusion

Clinical signs: Anorexia, poor grooming, or lack of coprophagy. These lead to projection of the lower incisors out of the mouth and impingement of the upper incisors into the hard palate (Figure 13.7). Molar malocclusion and overgrowth will also produce a more open position of the jaw at rest and so lead to incisor malocclusion.

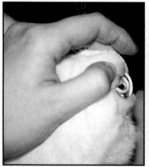 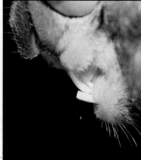

Figure 13.7: Incisor malocclusion.

Treatment: See Tooth trimming and Incisor removal.

Molar malocclusion

Loss of an opposing tooth may lead to overgrowth due to lack of attrition. Fractures of the skull, neoplasia, osteomyelitis and iatrogenic trauma may also lead to malocclusion of the cheek teeth and subsequent dental problems. An acquired condition is thought to be due to lack of wear. Rabbits in captivity are fed highly concentrated feeds rather than grazing a natural abrasive food for hours each day. The molars continue to grow, and if not adequately worn down, excessive enamel spurs develop on the crowns (causing intraoral soft tissue injury) and root overgrowth (causing bone pain). As the extending root penetrates the jaw, the alveolar bulla perforates; the condition is now irreversible (Figure 13.8). The associated stretching of the exposed periosteum causes chronic pain. The animal will often react adversely when the apical areas are palpated. Elongated molar roots or (more commonly) incisor root pathology may impinge on the nasolacrimal duct leading to lacrimation or dacryocystitis (infection of the nasolacrimal duct). The condition may progress to periodontal infection, tooth root abscessation and osteomyelitis.

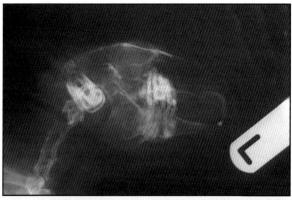

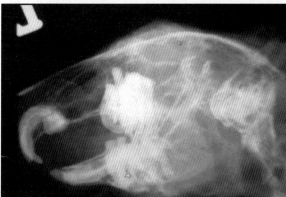

Fig 13.8: Radiographs showing advanced dental disease; note overgrowth of roots and penetration of the mandibular cortex.

Clinical signs: Anorexia, weight loss, excessive salivation, difficulty in prehension, mastication and swallowing may be observed if the tongue and cheeks are lacerated by dental spurs. Signs of pain, e.g. bruxism (grinding), aggression, lethargy may be seen associated with dental disease and oral soft tissue damage. If abscessation of the tooth root has occurred the rabbit will present with facial swelling.

Treatment: Analgesia may assist in the care of these animals and improve appetite but no true cure is possible. If the alveolar bulla is intact, coronal reduction may arrest the root elongation and allow the periapical tissues to recover. As the teeth come back into wear, an abrasive diet is offered to encourage normal tooth wear. The rabbit should be weighed at least weekly and skull radiography used to monitor the condition.

Incisor tooth fracture

Clinical signs
There is a history of trauma (iatrogenic or from a fall), anorexia and weight loss.

Treatment
The rabbit should be given appropriate antibiosis and analgesia. The exposed pulp tissue should be treated aseptically. A partial pulpectomy and application of calcium hydroxide cement may be used to seal the defect. The opposing tooth will require corrective trimming until the damaged tooth comes into wear. If the periapical tissues have been damaged, the tooth may fail to regrow and the opposing tooth will require regular trimming.

Miscellaneous conditions

Step mouth
The cheek teeth may wear at different rates leading to an irregular occlusal surface across the cheek teeth. Poor mineralization has been suggested as a causative factor. If neither lateral tipping of the tooth nor root elongation have occurred, the condition may be treated by coronal reduction, as previously described, and the introduction of an abrasive diet.

Caries

Clinical signs:

- Increased radiolucency of crown
- Soft dental tissue on probing
- Food impaction between teeth and poorly mineralized teeth.

Treatment:

- Dietary correction to minimize sugary substances and increase abrasive dietary constituents
- Occlusal correction.

Periodontal disease

Clinical signs:

- Halitosis
- Food impaction
- Facial abscessation.

Aetiology: The periodontal ligaments of continuously erupting teeth are relatively wide, and easily damaged by impacted food and infection. Infection may spread to the root apex and result in osteomyelitis.

Diagnostic approach and treatment: Radiography is used to investigate the extent of the periodontal disease. Extraction of the infected tooth is required to effect a cure. Curettage of the infected socket and bone followed by lavage of the abscess cavity is required. The cavity is then packed with calcium hydroxide and left open to granulate.

DENTAL SURGERY PROCEDURES

Tooth trimming

The use of nail clippers or wire cutters is not recommended for trimming teeth for the following reasons:

- The excessive force applied to the crown as it is cut may damage the periapical germinal tissues, adversely affecting future tooth growth
- Longitudinal fissures in the tooth may be produced. These may lead to periodontal problems and pulp infection
- Accurate reshaping and smoothing of the teeth is difficult, if not impossible
- The sharp edges created may lacerate the tongue and cheeks or contribute to oral discomfort.

A burr in a dental handpiece should be used for accurate and humane tooth trimming and shaping (Figure 13.9). The pulp cavity normally extends to approximately half the length of the normal occlusal height of the tooth, i.e. midway between normal height and the gingival margin. Trimming and reshaping to normal height should not therefore expose the pulp cavity. Many rabbits will tolerate trimming of the incisors while conscious and manually restrained. A tongue depressor or syringe case of appropriate size should be placed behind the incisors to protect the soft tissues while trimming.

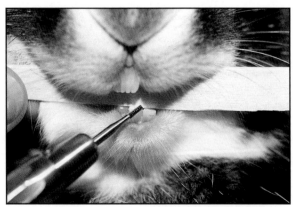

Figure 13.9: *Trimming incisors using a handheld burr.*

In order to examine the oral cavity fully for corrective trimming of the molars, a general anaesthetic is necessary to abolish chewing and tongue movements and allow manipulation of the mouth and tongue. An appropriately sized guard is used to retract and protect the soft tissues either side of the tooth to be burred. The affected molar is burred down and reshaped. Each tooth should not be subjected to long periods of burring that may produce excessive heat and damage the pulp tissue. The debris should be wiped away frequently. Ideally, the animal should have an endotracheal tube placed for the supply of oxygen and/or anaesthetic gases, and to prevent inhalation of the tooth debris.

Damage to the soft tissues should be treated appropriately by flushing or cleaning with dilute chlorhexidine and systemic antibiotic therapy instigated if the lesions are infected. The short-term use of an oral topical anaesthetic gel may give some relief from oral discomfort while the soft tissues heal or an NSAID may be administered for 24–48 hours.

Incisor removal

Indications

- Incisor malocclusion
- Tooth root infection
- Loss of opposing tooth.

Many owners may have the impression that, following removal of the incisor teeth, the rabbit will not require any further treatment. This may not always be the case. However, although it may not be possible to cure the rabbit's dental disease if the molars also require regular therapy, incisor removal may alleviate the clinical problem to some extent by enabling the rabbit to eat more easily. Maloccluded incisors are usually no longer functional, and merely serve as a obstruction to feeding. The lips prehend the food and the cheek teeth grind the food so in most instances a normal diet can be fed after incisor removal, although larger items, e.g. carrots require grating.

Surgical technique

Radiography is required before incisor removal, to establish any associated pathology and molar involvement. This is essential to evaluate the dental disease associated with the premolars and molars as well as the incisors.

1. The gingival attachment around the tooth is cut using a proprietary elevator, a blunted needle or a no. 11 scalpel blade. The periodontal ligament should be elevated all around the tooth. Ensure the elevator follows the line of the tooth, taking into account the natural curvature of the tooth. The ligament is strongest on the medial and lateral sides of the tooth.

2. Once elevated, the tooth is extracted using gentle traction. Excessive traction to extract the teeth may result in fracture of the teeth, especially if they are of poor quality (Figure 13.10). It is wise to attempt extraction using the fingers rather than instruments to produce less traction.

   If a tooth breaks, the rabbit must be re-presented a few weeks later when the crowns have erupted for completion of the extraction. If the periapical tissues have been damaged, regrowth may not occur and surgery may be required to retrieve the stump before it serves as a nidus for infection or progresses to tooth root abscessation.
3. As the incisor teeth are removed they should be gently rotated and pressed into the socket before extraction to destroy germinal tissue and prevent regrowth.
4. The sockets may be packed with an anticoagulant sponge to limit haemorrhage in the postoperative period.

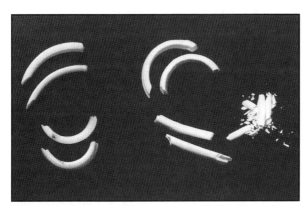

Figure 13.10: Extracted incisors – note the fragility and poor quality of the teeth from some rabbits, which makes removal difficult.

Postoperative considerations

Analgesia must be provided in the postoperative period. The animals should be bright, alert and eating within 2 hours postoperatively following appropriate anaesthesia and with appropriate analgesia.

If substantial soft tissue or bone trauma was associated with this condition (or created iatrogenically), then a nasogastric tube may be used for nutritional supplementation until the rabbit is able to eat normally (see Chapter 1). The animal should be weighed daily in the postoperative period to ensure weight loss does not occur. Food items must be prepared in bite-sized particles; vegetables may need to be chopped or grated. If the animal does not eat voluntarily within 24 hours, nutritional and fluid support must be instigated and the cause of the anorexia investigated.

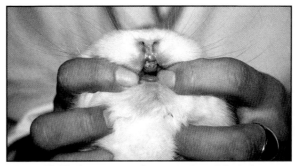

Figure 13.11: Appearance after extraction of the incisors.

The normal rabbit uses the incisors for grooming: the rabbit should therefore be groomed regularly by the owner to prevent matting of the coat.

The appearance of the rabbit following incisor extraction is shown in Figure 13.11.

Molar extraction

Some abnormal molars may be extracted per os by simple traction if the periodontal ligament is weak or root pathology is such that the tooth is loose. The curvature of the tooth should be taken into account when attempting to extract it. If the periodontal ligament is still intact, it may be broken down using a modified elevator and the tooth extracted orally. The small size of the oral cavity relative to the instrument makes intraoral manipulation of the tooth difficult.

The removal of a molar via a buccotomy incision, removal of alveolar bone and replacement of a gingival flap requires careful technique and intensive postoperative care to ensure a successful recovery.

Each molar opposes with two others. These teeth may need corrective trimming following extraction of one opposing tooth, and so the rabbit should be checked regularly.

REFERENCES AND FURTHER READING

Brown SA (1992) Surgical removal of incisors in the rabbit. *Journal of Small Animal Exotic Medicine* **1**, 150–153

Crossley DA (1995) Clinical aspects of lagomorph dental anatomy: the rabbit (*Oryctolagus cuniculus*). *Journal of Veterinary Dentistry* **12**, 137–140

DeSanto J (1997) Hypertrophic osteopathy associated with an intrathoracic neoplasm in a rabbit. *Journal of the American Veterinary Medical Association* **210**, 1322–1323

Flecknell PA (1998) Developments in the veterinary care of rabbits and rodents. *In Practice* **20**, 286–295

Gorrel C (1996) Teeth trimming in rabbits and rodents (letter). *Veterinary Record*, Nov. 23, 528

Harcourt-Brown F (1997) Diagnosis, treatment and prognosis of dental disease in pet rabbits. *In Practice* **19**, 407–421

Jenkins J (1997) Surgery of rabbits. In: Proceedings of the House Rabbit Society Veterinary Conference, pp.95–108

Lobprise HB (1991) Dental and oral disease in lagomorphs. *Journal of Veterinary Dentistry* **8**(2), 11–17

CHAPTER FOURTEEN

Euthanasia

Sally O. Walshaw

INTRODUCTION

The attachment that rabbit owners feel toward their rabbit companions is as intense as that felt by owners of dogs and cats (Figure 14.1). With their round heads, large eyes, and soft fur, rabbits bring out the nurturing side of people. In addition, the frisky behaviour of a house rabbit brings great joy to the owners. The role of the veterinary surgeon and veterinary nurse at the time of euthanasia is to provide a peaceful death for the animal and to comfort the owner. It is important to remember what is lost when a pet dies. The owner loses a companion and non-judgemental love object, a chance for play, an opportunity for responsibility, and a link to the natural world. Psychologists and others acknowledge that loving animals can be good for people, and that it is normal for owners to experience sadness when a pet dies. Grief is the price we pay for love.

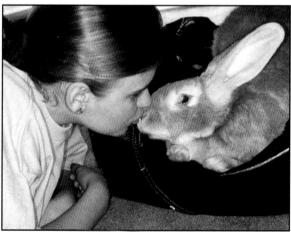

Figure 14.1: Rabbit with owner.

EUTHANASIA: GENERAL PRINCIPLES

Veterinary surgery policies

Establishing policies that will ensure a peaceful death for the animal and a degree of comfort for the owner takes planning. A scheduled euthanasia should be performed in a quiet room, out of the surgery 'high traffic' areas, and at a quiet time in the surgery's schedule. Standard procedures may include a team

approach, a tranquillizing agent, an intravenous catheter, and arrangements for the owner to be present during euthanasia. All surgery personnel who assist with euthanasia during regular or emergency hours should be familiar with the clinic's billing policy for this procedure. Surgery euthanasia policy should address such issues as the circumstances under which a rabbit will be euthanased in its own home. Follow-up communication with the owner, in a few days and after a few weeks, is very much appreciated. Finally, a support system is important for veterinary surgery workers because performing euthanasia and consoling bereaved clients can be emotionally exhausting.

Communication with the owner

A survey of animal owners on the subject of euthanasia, conducted by veterinary students at Michigan State University in 1996, revealed confusion and concern over details of the euthanasia process. Many owners assumed that euthanasia itself (not just the injection) was inherently painful for the animal. Some believed that the animal is fully conscious with a paralysed respiratory system. They were especially upset if they had witnessed an animal euthanasia that involved struggling or strong restraint methods. Some owners were shocked at how quickly death occurred after the injection was given; they expected a slow slumber-like process. Owners had abundant praise for veterinary surgeons when the procedure went smoothly, when the veterinary surgeon and veterinary nurse exhibited compassion toward the animal and the people, and when the owners were adequately prepared for what would happen.

General considerations for euthanasia

When striving to provide a peaceful death for a rabbit, one must minimize the stress factors for the species and for the particular rabbit. For all animals, common stress factors at the time of euthanasia may include a new setting and unfamiliar people. Some veterinary surgery workers have a rapport with rabbits and, ideally, they should be included on the euthanasia team. Another stress factor for a rabbit is a slippery examination table, so a towel or blanket should be available.

Tranquillizers

The temperament of an individual rabbit is also a factor. The fearful or aggressive rabbit may be a difficult patient, but it, too, deserves a peaceful death. Use of a tranquillizing agent, such as acepromazine maleate (0.7–1.5 mg/kg s.c.) is a humane approach for all rabbits. Alternatively, medetomidine (0.25 mg/kg s.c.) produces marked sedation and moderate analgesia, and has a more rapid onset of action than acepromazine. It does, however, produce peripheral vasoconstriction which makes placement of an intravenous catheter more difficult. Acepromazine (0.5 mg/kg) mixed with butorphanol (0.1 mg/kg), given subcutaneously, produces marked sedation, peripheral vasodilation and some analgesia, and even more profound analgesia is provided by a mixture of fentanyl and fluanisone ('Hypnorm', Janssen, 0.3 ml/kg s.c.). The tranquillizer or sedative will relax the rabbit and give the owner a few minutes to 'say goodbye' before the injection of the euthanasia agent.

Euthanasia

The owner who chooses to be present during euthanasia probably prefers that the rabbit remains conscious until the euthanasia agent is administered. In the opinion of this author, however, the most peaceful painless method of rabbit euthanasia, especially for a fearful or aggressive rabbit, begins with a subcutaneous injection of an anaesthetic agent. An example of a subcutaneous combination for pre-euthanasia anaesthesia, is ketamine (35 mg/kg) and xylazine (7 mg/kg) (see also Chapter 12).

After the injection, the rabbit can continue to eat some favourite treats while it gradually loses consciousness over 7 to 10 minutes. When the rabbit is recumbent, the euthanasia agent is injected.

The rabbit's physical condition will determine the method of euthanasia in some cases. If an animal is very tiny, dehydrated, or in hypovolaemic shock, finding a suitable vein may be very difficult or even impossible. In such cases, euthanasia may consist of an intraperitoneal injection of a barbiturate anaesthetic agent such as pentobarbitone (90–120 mg/kg). If necessary, once the rabbit is anaesthetized, additional injectable euthanasia agents may be administered via intracardiac injection.

The age of the rabbit is an important consideration in some cases. Very young animals tend to wiggle and may react in unexpected ways to euthanasia agents. Elderly animals have fragile skin and veins, so care must be taken when clipping hair or inserting a needle into a vein.

There are several other factors to be considered when planning euthanasia. The owners may have preferences regarding euthanasia and burial of the rabbit. Surgery factors include the available euthanasia agents and equipment. In addition, training of surgery personnel in euthanasia procedures will minimize stress for the animal and ensure the safety of everyone present.

EMERGENCY EUTHANASIA

In cases of emergency euthanasia, two important additional factors must be taken into account: first, the animal is often in pain, in shock, or in great distress; and, secondly, the owners may be in emotional turmoil with feelings of anger, shock, denial and guilt.

If the owners and the veterinary surgeon agree that euthanasia is indicated, the veterinary surgeon should explain to the rabbit's owners what will take place. The owners need to know that the surgery team will work quickly to relieve the animal's pain. Furthermore, after the animal has been euthanased, the veterinary surgeon or nurse must take time to talk with the owners. As with other owners whose rabbits have died or been euthanased, follow-up telephone calls during the next few weeks will be very much appreciated. The conversation can begin with a surgery staff member saying, 'Hello, we were just thinking about you and wondering how you are getting on'. If the owner seems to be having a difficult time, the staff member can provide information on pet loss support counselling.

SCHEDULED EUTHANASIA

When scheduling an appointment for a rabbit's euthanasia, the surgery staff member should discuss various options with the owner. Options include owner-present euthanasia, later viewing of the rabbit's body by children or other family members, and arrangements for the disposal of the rabbit's body.

The euthanasia appointment is scheduled for a typically quiet time at the surgery. A towel or blanket should be available in the room for the rabbit. Surgery staff members should talk to the rabbit with affection and gentleness; these are the last few minutes of the rabbit's life. The veterinary surgeon or veterinary nurse explains the euthanasia method and how it produces death. The owner needs to know that once the actual injection begins, the rabbit will die very quickly. By using a tranquillizer before the euthanasia agent, the possibility of involuntary movements or muscle spasms is minimized, but owners should be informed that this could occur.

If the owner elects to be present during the actual euthanasia, it is best to take the rabbit away from them briefly. The veterinary surgeon should explain that the rabbit will be taken to a quiet treatment area with good lighting for placing an intravenous catheter and for administering a tranquillizer (Figure 14.2). The catheter should be bandaged neatly in place (Figure 14.3) and the rabbit returned to the owner. The owner can then have a few minutes to comfort the rabbit and to make this an occasion for affection and peacefulness.

When the owner indicates that it is time to perform euthanasia, the veterinary surgeon should ask if the owner would prefer to leave the room during the

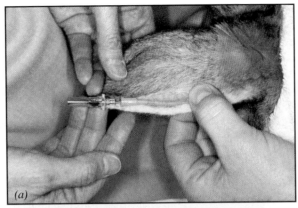

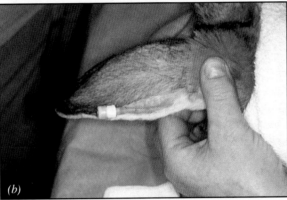

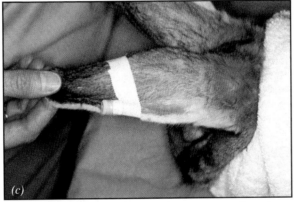

Figure 14.2: Inserting a 24 gauge intravenous catheter into a rabbit's marginal ear vein.

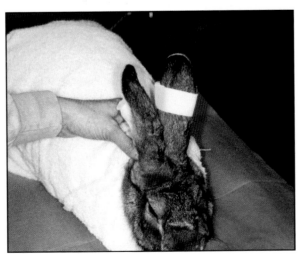

Figure 14.3: Rabbit wrapped in a towel with intravenous catheter taped in place.

injection of the euthanasia agent. The person holding the rabbit during the euthanasia injection has the task of thinking beautiful thoughts. Although animals do not read minds, they are masters of reading body language. This step may help soothe the animal in the last moments of its life.

After the rabbit has died, the surgery staff should allow the owner to spend time with the body. Providing tissues and a cool drink of water are gestures of kindness in this situation. If possible, surgery staff members can help the grieving owners by allowing them to leave the hospital by a private exit, rather than through a crowded waiting room.

PREPARING AN ANIMAL'S BODY FOR A VISIT BY THE OWNERS

The rabbit may die or be euthanased in the surgery without the owner or some other family members being present. It is not recommended for small children to be present during animal euthanasia. Children under the age of 12 years may have disturbing dreams after watching animal euthanasia and may fear injections and anaesthesia if, at a later date, they require these procedures themselves.

The rabbit's body should be placed on absorbent pads, in case of urine leaks, in a quiet room on a table or in an aesthetically pleasing box. Towels should be draped under and over the rabbit's body so that the head and shoulders are exposed. Glue will hold the eyelids closed if desired. Small flowers can be provided for the owner(s) to place on the rabbit's body. The veterinary surgeon and other surgery staff members should talk to the owners about their special rabbit and give them plenty of time to say goodbye.

CONSOLING BEREAVED CLIENTS

Attachments to animals and emotion over their deaths are striking examples of compassion and empathy among animal owners and members of the veterinary health care team. Compassion and empathy are some of our best human traits and allow us to care for and nurture each other, as well as animals.

Factors affecting grief
The circumstances of the death have a strong impact on grief. A sudden or traumatic death is a shock for the owner; therefore, such characteristics of grief as denial and anger may be exaggerated. This does not imply that an anticipated death of an aged rabbit is easy for the owner. However, the owner of a chronically ill rabbit may have been able to provide some special treats and comforting measures in the last days or weeks of the rabbit's life. Euthanasia of the rabbit may lead to some uneasiness later in the owner: he or she

may worry that the rabbit might have recovered from the illness or injury or, conversely, that the rabbit suffered due to the owner's delay in making the decision to euthanase.

The relationship of the person to the rabbit is another important factor affecting grief. Some members of a household have stronger attachments than others to an animal, and their grief may not get much support. Situations in which the rabbit was rescued from an animal shelter or nursed through an illness lead to exceptionally strong human–animal bonds and profound grief at the animal's death.

Other factors that may add to the burden of grief at a rabbit's death are recent illness or death of other significant individuals, or other major losses in the grieving person's life. Stress and isolation can intensify the normal grief reaction in an owner when a companion animal dies.

Grief in adults

John Schneider (1984) wrote, 'Grief is a process of discovering the extent of what was lost and the subsequent process of discovering the extent of what was *not* lost or what can now take place.' A grieving individual may experience some or all of the characteristics in a variable order and for a variable length of time. The commonly listed characteristics are denial, weeping, bodily distress, anger, guilt, and loss of pattern of conduct. All the characteristics of grief are considered normal by psychologists but they seem 'crazy' to the individual experiencing them. It is normal for a person experiencing a significant loss to take more time than usual to do ordinary or routine tasks. Doubting one's own sanity during this period of confusion only adds to the pain experienced.

Grieving takes at least one full year after a significant loss. A number of tasks await the grieving person. In the first stage, aimed at limiting awareness, the grieving person alternates between holding on to positive memories and diminishing the loss by focusing on negative aspects. The second stage involves gaining awareness and perspective. During this stage, the grieving individual faces his or her own mortality and enters a time of healing. The person may spend time in quiet reflection.

The ultimate goal is growth from bereavement. The outcome is ideally more than just acceptance of the loss but an enhancement of such qualities as openness, empathy, wisdom, strength and joy.

Grief in children

A child's understanding of grief is influenced by the child's age and life experiences. Children under 3 years of age react to separation but have little or no concept of death. Between the ages of 3 and 5 years, children see death as immobility or as a departure but they may believe that death is reversible. Children expect parents to 'mend' dead things. Children at this age also may believe in magical concepts. The young

child may think that 'I wished the animal was dead because it chewed up my favourite toy and the wish caused the animal's death.' Children of 6 to 9 years begin to understand that everything will die, but they also may associate death with darkness and violence. It is normal for children in this age group to ask what happens to dead bodies and even to suggest digging up a pet's body. Older children and young adults may fear death's unpredictability and they may feel responsible for an animal's death.

A young child's grief is somewhat different from the adult experience. Young children (less than 10 years of age) have a shorter sadness span; they grieve intensely but they may interrupt their grief with play and then return to the subject later. Young children have strong tendencies to deny that death has occurred. The young child tends to avoid behaviour that might result in rejection by the parents, so a child will talk about grief only if the parent seems comfortable with the subject. Another normal aspect of grief in children is the reactivation of the subject of a specific death as their physical and mental growth initiates developmental changes.

Complicated grief

Complicated grief may manifest itself in a number of ways. There are different types of complicated grief, including absent, distorted, converted or chronic. Grief that seems to be absent after a person has suffered a major loss is actually delayed mourning. In distorted grief, the individual feels only anger or guilt and has difficulty moving through other stages of the grief experience. Converted grief occurs when the person avoids the mourning process by activities like overeating, substance abuse, and overworking. In chronic grief, the person focuses intensely on the dead individual, as if to keep the dead alive.

The negative consequences of uncompleted grieving are significant. It is less likely that the person will resolve subsequent losses, and the individual's energy is kept bound to the loss and to the past. The person is likely to suffer low-level constant depression. Multiple illnesses, chronic fatigue, irritability, decreased interest and pleasure in work and life, concentration problems, sleeping and eating disorders, restlessness, and insensitivity or indifference to others all characterize incomplete grieving.

Consoling bereaved adults

It is important for members of the veterinary health care team to comfort the owner by acknowledging the significance of the loss of the rabbit. Few people outside the immediate family will understand grief over the loss of any animal, especially a non-traditional house pet such as a rabbit. We can support the normality of grief by recognizing such components as denial, weeping, bodily distress, anger, guilt, and the loss of pattern of conduct. Knowing the signs of complicated grief will enable the veterinary team members to suggest support systems that might be beneficial for a particular owner.

One way we can help grieving owners is to encourage them to talk about the rabbit, at the time of euthanasia and a week or two later by telephone. It is normal for grieving people to search for meaning by talking about their losses repeatedly; this reviewing process is essential for mourning a significant loss. Most clients really appreciate continued comforting measures. Surgery staff members can send a sympathy card, telephone the owner, or donate to a charitable organization in memory of the rabbit.

Consoling bereaved children

Parents and friends can comfort the grieving child with empathy, love and understanding. Sometimes parents are distraught at a child's tears when a pet dies. A major role of a parent, from the moment of the child's birth, is to respond quickly to a crying child. However, even for a child, grief is normal and cannot be instantly soothed as with other sources of a child's sadness. Psychologists point out that a child who experiences grief within the context of a loving family gains preparation for many difficult life situations.

The veterinary surgeon and other clinic staff can help parents with a child's grief in a number of ways. Parents can be assured the child is welcome at the surgery to see the rabbit's body. Surgery team members can offer comforting words to the child if present. The veterinary surgery can provide a list of books dealing with children's grief or even keep some books and pamphlets on hand for loaning to owners. Children benefit from receiving information essential to their understanding of death. A young child needs to know a definition and cause of death, such as, 'Your rabbit died because he was very old and his heart could not keep working'. The grieving child needs to know that it is normal to feel anger, sadness and even guilt. Parents can also provide a religious or philosophical framework about death for the child, e.g. heaven or natural cycles.

Some special questions may arise with regard to handling grief in a child. If parents ask whether it is best to lie about the circumstances of an animal's death to a child, the answer is no. If the child discovered that a parent had lied about such an important subject, trust in the parent might be shattered. When trying to understand the death of a pet, the child may ask the parent, 'Will you die?' An honest, but reassuring answer is 'Yes, but not for a long time'.

COPING IN THE VETERINARY SURGERY

It is important for veterinary surgery workers to discuss euthanasia cases, especially if there were exceptionally emotional issues involved. Losing a

favourite patient or consoling a bereaved client can be exhausting and staff members deserve comforting measures too.

To choose appropriate ways of comforting each other, veterinary surgery workers should think about how other people have helped them in times of grief. It is important to support the expression of feelings. Rituals, like a moment of silence, or a walk outdoors, can confirm the dignity of the person and of the animal. A photo scrapbook of hospital patients with tributes written by owners and staff members is a way of remembering the joy a rabbit can bring (Figure 14.4).

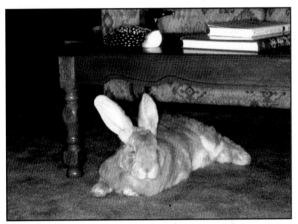

Figure 14.4: *Photographs can bring back fond memories.*

CONCLUSION

Veterinary medicine has been called both a science and an art. This is especially true with euthanasia. There are many methods and drugs that are effective; the individual veterinary surgeon must develop and modify procedures for each situation that are both humane for the animal and acceptable to its owners. There is comfort in knowing that euthanasia is the last kind thing we can do for an animal.

Finally, many grieving rabbit owners have sent tributes and photos to house rabbit journals and to pet loss sites on the computer-accessible World Wide Web. Euthanasia of a beloved rabbit is a very sorrowful time for the owner.

REFERENCES AND FURTHER READING

Buscaglia L (1982) *The Fall of Freddie the Leaf*. Holt, Rinehart, and Winston, New York (Children's book)
Grollman E (1967) *Explaining Death to Children*. Beacon Press, Boston
Hart LA and Hart BL (1987) Grief and stress from so many animal deaths. *Companion Animal Practice*. **1,** (1) March issue, 20-27
Katcher AH and Beck AM (1983) *New Perspectives on Our Lives with Companion Animals*. University of Pennsylvania Press, Philadelphia
Katcher AH and Rosenberg MA (1979) Euthanasia and the management of the client's grief. *Compendium on Continuing Education for the Practising Veterinarian* **1,** 887-891

Kay WJ, Nieburg HA, Kutscher AH, Grey RM and Fudin CE, (eds) (1984) *Pet Loss and Human Bereavement.* Iowa State University Press, Ames

Kubler-Ross E (1969) *On Death and Dying.* Macmillan, New York.

Lagoni L, Butler C and Hetts S (1994) *The Human–Animal Bond and Grief.* WC Saunders, Philadelphia

Madewell BR (1981) Interaction with owners of cancer-stricken pets. *Journal of the American Veterinary Medical Association* **178,** 30–32

McNicholas J and Collis GM (1995) The end of a relationship: coping with pet loss. In: *The Waltham Book of Human–Animal Interaction: Benefits and Responsibilities of Pet Ownership,* ed. I Robinson, pp. 127–143. Elsevier Science, Oxford

Nieburg HA and Fischer A (1982) *Pet Loss – A Thoughtful Guide for Adults and Children.* Harper & Row, New York

Randolph JW (1994) Learning from your own pet's euthanasia. *Journal of the American Veterinary Medical Association* **205,** 544–545

Rogers F (1988) *When a Pet Dies.* Putnam's Sons, New York (Children's book)

Schneider J (1984) *Stress, Loss, and Grief.* University Park Press, Baltimore

Stewart M, Docherty A and Brown A (1996) *When a Pet Dies: A learning pack for people who support owners when their pet dies.* Society for Companion Animal Studies, Callender, Scotland

Viorst J (1971) *The Tenth Good Thing about Barney.* Atheneum, Hartford, Connecticut (Children's book)

White EB (1952) *Charlotte's Web.* Dell, New York (Children's book)

Williams M (1983) *The Velveteen Rabbit.* Simon and Schuster, New York (Children's book)

Wolfelt AD (1991) *A Child's View of Grief.* Center for Loss and Life Transition, Fort Collins, Colorado

Wolfelt AD (1992) *Understanding Grief: Helping Yourself Heal.* Accelerated Development Publishers, Muncie, Indiana

Index